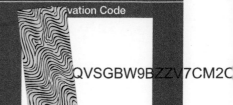

PHARMACY **OSCES**
AND COMPETENCY-BASED
ASSESSMENTS

PHARMACY **OSCES** AND COMPETENCY-BASED ASSESSMENTS

Sharon Haughey BSc PhD MPSNI FFRPS
Senior Lecturer
School of Pharmacy
Queen's University
Belfast
Northern Ireland
UK

Roisín O'Hare BSc MSc DPharm MPSNI(IP) FFRPS
Lead Teacher Practitioner
Pharmacist
Northern Ireland University Network
Craigavon Area Hospital
Portadown, Northern Ireland, UK

For additional online content visit StudentConsult.com

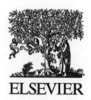

ELSEVIER

Edinburgh London New York Oxford Philadelphia St Louis Sydney Toronto

ELSEVIER

Notices

Knowledge and best practice in this field are constantly changing. As new research and experience broaden our understanding, changes in research methods, professional practices, or medical treatment may become necessary.

Practitioners and researchers must always rely on their own experience and knowledge in evaluating and using any information, methods, compounds, or experiments described herein. In using such information or methods they should be mindful of their own safety and the safety of others, including parties for whom they have a professional responsibility.

With respect to any drug or pharmaceutical products identified, readers are advised to check the most current information provided (i) on procedures featured or (ii) by the manufacturer of each product to be administered, to verify the recommended dose or formula, the method and duration of administration, and contraindications. It is the responsibility of practitioners, relying on their own experience and knowledge of their patients, to make diagnoses, to determine dosages and the best treatment for each individual patient, and to take all appropriate safety precautions.

To the fullest extent of the law, neither the Publisher nor the authors, contributors, or editors, assume any liability for any injury and/or damage to persons or property as a matter of products liability, negligence or otherwise, or from any use or operation of any methods, products, instructions, or ideas contained in the material herein.

ISBN: 978-0-7020-6701-3

Content Strategist: Pauline Graham
Content Development Specialist: Carole McMurray
Project Manager: Julie Taylor
Design: Miles Hitchen
Illustration Manager: Karen Giacomucci, Amy Naylor

Contents

Contents

Foreword

A decade ago, few (if any) pharmacy students knew what the acronym 'OSCE' denoted. Few (if any) educators used competency – based assessments to guide teaching, learning, and evaluation. Few (if any) pharmacists were taught or tested in the area of clinical skills.

Today, the practice of pharmacy has changed significantly. Pharmacists work in collaborative, interprofessional settings with other health care providers, delivering high quality patient-focused care and services. The activities of pharmacists have shifted away from dispensing and inventory stewardship towards a patient – facing role involving direct provision of information, guidance and clinical services to those in need of care. Pharmacy educators around the globe have led this evolution, and each year, new graduates from pharmacy degree programs enter a profession rapidly changing to meet the needs of their health care system.

Historically, pharmacists have been mainly concerned with the safe dispensing of quality medicines: in this environment, pharmacists' work could be judged in a binary manner (either 'right' or 'wrong'). Pharmacy education of this era was focused on technical skills associated with compounding and dispensing, as the opportunity for pharmacists to independently exercise professional judgement was somewhat limited. Today, as pharmacists' roles and responsibilities have expanded and pharmacy technicians are playing a more prominent independent role on the dispensing side of the operation, pharmacists work is less clear cut, and less amenable to 'right' or 'wrong' judgments. Pharmacists must manage complex medical, pharmacotherapeutic, economic, and psycho-social issues in their day-to-day work, requiring them to integrate diverse bodies of knowledge, leverage existing and develop new skills, and ultimately take greater responsibility for the clinical and therapeutic decisions they make. In this environment, pharmacy education has evolved significantly to help new graduates develop the confidence they need to assume new responsibilities fully and effectively. With this evolution in education, there has been a growing awareness of the need for and value of different assessment models to assure students, their teachers, professionals and most importantly patients that pharmacists are ready, willing, and able to provide them with the care they need.

Competency – based assessment models have evolved as the standard in most health professional education programs around the world. These models reconceptualize the education of health professionals as the acquisition of knowledge, skills, and attitudes that allow students to confidently meet diverse real-world health care challenges and situations. Historically, education of professionals was built on the assumption that if students 'know' they can automatically translate that knowledge into 'doing' or action. Competency-based assessment challenges that traditional view of education and uses diverse methods to provide all stakeholders with assurances that professionals can actually apply what they have learned in a real world context in a safe and effective manner.

Competency – based assessments tend to focus on the performance of a professional role within a controlled and supervised setting, allowing the student to gain feedback and learn from the experience while giving the educator an opportunity to understand how theory gets translated into practice. Within many health professions, the objective structured clinical examination – or OSCE – has emerged as a primary tool for competency-based assessment.

When well designed and properly administered, OSCEs have a demonstrated track record of success in providing reliable, valid, defensible and generalizable results regarding individual student's readiness for the responsibilities for day-to-day professional practice.

OSCEs have been used for many decades in fields such as medicine, and medical educators have pioneered and refined methods for case development, exam administration, and analysis of results that provide invaluable guidance to pharmacy educators. The context of pharmacy education and practice is different than medicine, and pharmacists' reliance on communication (listening, speaking, observing) as a core clinical skill is arguably higher than it is for other 'touching' professions such as medicine or nursing. As a result, pharmacy OSCEs have evolved in unique ways that reflect the reality and context of the pharmacy profession itself – building upon the experience and tradition of other professions but adapting these to the needs of pharmacy students and pharmacists.

Today, OSCEs are a widely used competency-based assessment method in pharmacy around the world. In Canada, the entry-to-practice registration examination for all pharmacists seeking licensure in that country involves a 16-station OSCE. In New Zealand, the OSCE has emerged as an integral part of the pre-registration assessment process for new pharmacists. Across the United States, many pharmacy degree programs have incorporated OSCEs into their curricula, as a tool for both program evaluation and for providing students with direct and practical feedback on their readiness for practice.

Across the United Kingdom and Ireland, OSCEs are used in a diverse array of contexts in both professional education and in continuing professional development. There is significant flexibility possible within the OSCE framework, and this flexibility allows for a high degree of customization to the learner's context. As a result, for some students, OSCEs may appear bewildering, mysterious, or simply frightening.

The authors of this reference are to be congratulated for developing a useful, practical and informative guide to demystifying the OSCE process for students, pharmacists, educators, and the general public. In the chapters that follow, you will see how well constructed OSCEs are indeed a unique and invaluable form of assessment and that when understood in this light they are nothing to fear. The authors' first hand experiences in actually developing and administering OSCEs provides them with unique insights into the process that they generously share with readers. Depending upon your interest in OSCEs, you will find something of value and importance to guide your preparation, practice, or professional development.

As the profession of pharmacy continues to evolve – and as pharmacy educators continue to actively contribute to and lead this process – references such as this will assume greater importance. In the pages ahead you will learn much about OSCEs and appreciate how valuable they are in helping all of us ensure the profession and its practitioners continue to serve the public in a safe and effective manner.

Zubin Austin BScPhm MBA MISc PhD
Professor and Murray Koffler Chair in Management
Academic Director – Centre for Practice Excellence
Leslie Dan Faculty of Pharmacy, University of Toronto, Canada

Preface

Prescribing medicines to a patient remains the most common intervention made by the National Health Service (www.england.nhs.uk).

Medicines are crucial for maintaining health, preventing illness, managing chronic conditions and treating acute diseases. Where medicines are not used optimally, patients can end up either not getting the intended benefit or, at worst, suffering adverse effects and in some cases being admitted to hospital.

Undergraduate pharmacy students are required to know how to make and administer medicines, design and deliver medicines as well as diagnose and optimally treat illnesses. Patient care and safety is paramount during the undergraduate degree and beyond into pharmacy practice.

Evaluations of the competence of healthcare professional students, including undergraduate pharmacists, using simulated assessments including Objective Structured Clinical Examinations (OSCEs) and Criterion Referenced Assessments (CRAs) are increasingly commonplace.

OSCEs and CRAs simulate aspects of real-life future pharmacy practice and provide undergraduate students with the opportunity to integrate their knowledge of medicinal chemistry, pharmaceutics, therapeutics, legislation as well as their clinical skills, numeracy, communication, and empathy in order to demonstrate their ability to provide safe and effective patient care.

In terms of employability, it is also important that the pharmacy student develops the ability to 'think on their feet'. Being able to make a decision, in a timely manner, which optimizes patient care is one of the key skills that employers ask for time and time again.

The aim of this book is therefore to provide a resource to support students to develop and practice these key skills. This book is designed as a useful resource for undergraduate students, clinical tutors and those involved in teaching students on an undergraduate pharmacy degree course.

Glossary

ACT: accuracy checking technician
BPM: beats per minute
COPD: chronic obstructive pulmonary disease
CRA: criterion referenced assessment
DoH: Department of Health
FEV$_1$: forced expiratory volume in one second
FVC: forced vital capacity
GOLD: Global Initiative for Chronic Obstructive Lung Disease
GPhC: General Pharmaceutical Council
GTN: glyceryl trinitrate
HCP: healthcare professional
HR: heart rate
IHD: ischaemic heart disease
INR: international normalized ratio
IV: intravenous
MDT: multidisciplinary team
MHRA: Medicines and Healthcare products Regulatory Agency

NHS: National Health Service
NPA: National Pharmacy Association
NPSA: National Patient Safety Agency
OSCE: objective structured clinical examination
OSPE: objective structure pharmacy examination
PEF: peak expiratory flow
PEFR: peak expiratory flow rate
PEG: percutaneous endoscopic gastrostomy
PIL: patient information leaflet
PMHx: patient medication history
PSNI: Pharmaceutical Society of Nothern Ireland
RPS: Royal Pharmaceutical Society
SHP: standardised healthcare professional
SOP: standard operating procedure
SP: standardized patient
SPC: summary of product characteristics
STEMI: ST elevation myocardial infarction

Acknowledgements

This book would not be possible without input from a wide variety of clinicians and academics, as well as pre-registration pharmacists, postgraduate and undergraduate students who have worked closely with us to shape the OSCEs and CRAs that you will practise in this book.

We would like to particularly thank all of the members of the Teacher Practitioner Team and the Pharmacy Practice Team at Queen's University Belfast including Dr Joanne Brown, Kathryn King, Sara Laird, Aine Liggett, Janet Magee, Fionnuala McCullagh, Niamh McGarry, Roisin McNulty, Fiona O'Neill, Louise Shephard, Johanne Barry, Alison Buchanan, Dr Maurice Hall, Dr Lezley-Anne Hanna, Fiona Hughes, Sharon McEvoy and Dr Carole Parsons.

We would also like to particularly thank all of the members of staff who were involved in the initial development and piloting of the criterion referenced assessments in the School of Pharmacy, Queen's University Belfast.

We would finally like to acknowledge the support and love of our understanding partners to whom we dedicate this book.

Introduction

Pharmacy is a 'regulated' profession; the General Pharmaceutical Council (GPhC) is the regulatory body for pharmacists and pharmacy technicians in England, Scotland and Wales and the Pharmaceutical Society of Northern Ireland (PSNI) is the professional leadership body and regulator for pharmacists in Northern Ireland. The regulator is responsible for ensuring that those pharmacists who attain status on the pharmaceutical register are appropriately trained initially and continue to participate in continuing education and professional development in order to maintain their position on the register.

Why do we need competency based assessments?

Recent events, including the Shipman Inquiry (Smith, 2002), the Elizabeth Lee case (Chemist & Druggist, 2010) and the Mid Staffordshire Public inquiry (Francis, 2013) support the growing public demand for heightened accountability from healthcare professionals, with an increasing emphasis on the attainment and maintenance of competence. The introduction of mandatory continuing professional development and the separation of the regulatory and professional leadership arms of the Royal Pharmaceutical Society of Great Britain (RPSGB) have occurred as a direct consequence of increased public and governmental scrutiny on the ability of the pharmacy profession to guarantee sustained competence from its members (DOH, 2006; DOH, 2007a; DOH, 2007b).

How is pharmacy as a profession evolving?

In the 1990s, the RPSGB launched a vision for pharmacy, known as 'Pharmacy in a New Age' or PIANA (RPSGB, 1996), to raise the profile of the profession and to demonstrate that pharmacists were not only prepared but are qualified to provide increasing contributions to the wider NHS agenda. PIANA was expanded in the 'Fit for the Future' programme (RPSGB, 2004a) which spearheaded improvements in pharmacy education including investment in research and development, the development of a pharmacy student code of conduct, fitness to practice systems as well as standards for education and training.

As with other healthcare professions, student assessment in pharmacy education has evolved over the past 20 years. Educators have struggled to adapt existing tools and develop novel evaluation methods which will estimate competence in a wide variety of clinical situations whilst remaining reliable, valid and lacking in subjectivity (Beck, Boh & O'Sullivan, 1995). The profession of pharmacy is increasingly expected to demonstrate the robustness of undergraduate pharmacy training and evidence of graduates' proficiency in upholding patient safety particularly with reference to high profile cases in the media where patient rights are paramount. In recognition of this, the GPhC launched guidelines for education and training

respondents (107/155) chose community volunteers followed by students, faculty and finally administrative staff. The community volunteers in this study also received the highest rating for the reality of their performance.

How do we ensure that this assessment is fair?

Fundamental aspects of every assessment include the ability to demonstrate the reliability and validity of the method as well as its objectivity. Many authors have investigated the psychometric properties in relation to the OSCE in a variety of diverse clinical fields. Healthcare education, both undergraduate and postgraduate, can be used to dynamically affect change in the behaviour of professional groups in real life practice. Use of OSCEs alone is unlikely to engender a sustained behavioural change, however, an alignment of teaching, learning as well as assessment in order to support clinical skills and performance would appear to have a greater chance at success (Hodges 2003a). The degree of validity of an assessment is a method of establishing that the evaluation reflects what it has been designed to measure (Corbo et al, 2006). An examination should measure what is intended (face validity) and include the assessment of relevant areas and skills representative of up-to-date clinical pharmacy practice (content validity) (Crossley, Humphries & Jolly, 2002; Turner & Dankowski, 2008).

Content validity is essential in any assessment. Educationalists describe the development of a blueprint or 'matrix' against which the content and competencies to be assessed during the examination are mapped to achieve content validity. The use of a blueprint also supports sufficient specification of examination contents as opposed to random topic selections. In order to maximise content validity, OSCE tasks are often developed by a team of clinical experts instead of one individual include an element of peer review and to provide a broader view of daily practice and pre-testing with student groups, and junior practitioners in the field of practice will help achieve face and content validity (Jeffries et al, 2007; Sturpe, 2010). Awaisu et al (2007), Hughes et al (2013) as well as Ragan, Virtue and Chi (2013) describe the use of a 'blueprint' for their station development and Awaisu et al (2007) explain how their station content was 'mapped' against the learning outcomes of the module. Evans et al (2011) delineate a robust authorship method where each new station developed has 4 versions, all of which are piloted, albeit with the authors, for feasibility of completion within the 5-minute timeframe. The use of standard setting either via borderline regression or the Angoff method was described by Awaisu et al (2010).

Another aspect of validity is the concept of 'contextual fidelity', that is, the importance of the *setting* in which the task is set and along what lines the student is expected to progress compared to content validity alone (Hodges 2003a). For example, taking a medication history from a patient who is blind would be an entirely different task from taking a medication history from a patient who does not have this disability and this 'context' will completely alter the approach that the student is trained to take and perhaps the level of success they will achieve.

An ideal evaluation tool should be objective and strive to remove assessor (and patient, if relevant) variability (Swanson & Norcini, 1989; Corbo et al, 2006). Assessor bias can result in differences in ratings given by the *same* assessor; that is, intra-rater variability. Differences between assessors can lead to inter-rater variability (Tamblyn et al, 1991). The reliability of an examination is its ability to differentiate consistently between ideal and poor performance in a reproducible manner. Due to the context specificity described previously in *How do we ensure that this assessment is fair?*, OSCEs require a large number of stations to enable examiners to determine student competence over a number of tasks with a number of different examiners. Quero Munoz (2005) in their high-stakes OSCE to facilitate pharmacy graduates entering the Canadian Pharmaceutical Register compared 26, 20 and 15 stations determining that 15 stations were sufficiently reliable for this type of assessment. For lower stakes undergraduate assessment, the number of stations reported in the studies evaluated varies from 3 (Hastings et al, 2010) to 17 (Evans et al, 2011).

What about feedback on OSCE performance?

Schultz et al (2004) found that the overwhelming majority of medical students questioned believed that feedback was essential for learning. OSCEs are valuable formative teaching tools, providing the opportunity for immediate feedback to students on performance as well as to teachers in relation to the level of student understanding of material delivered (Jeffries et al, 2007). Using OSCEs to inform both individual student learning as well as to expose areas of weakness in the course curriculum, or delivery, via student performance embeds the value of OSCEs as an integral aspect of the assessment program. Ragan, Virtue and Chi (2013) required candidates to complete a personal development plan to address the domains failed within their OSCE and Quero Munoz (2005) required a resit as their paper described registration with the Canadian Pharmaceutical Society.

OSCEs have been demonstrated to be objective, reliable (if sufficient stations are undertaken to determine reproducibility) and valid (if appropriate recognition of content and context are observed). It has been shown to be acceptable to students and lecturers as a fair method which demonstrates student ability in the practical aspects of the healthcare professions. It is also a feasible (if expensive and time-consuming) tool and the educational impact is undeniable, even without extensive feedback. In addition to an increased objectivity, advantages of OSCE are cited as an ability to control the complexity of the examination as well as the opportunity to provide feedback to students on their performance.

Challenges when preparing to implement an OSCE program include the cost of training academic staff to prepare and examine OSCEs as well as the training of standardised patients/doctors to adequately perform their roles. It is a huge organisational undertaking, usually requiring engagement from the entire academic team in order to examine all students in a timely manner. It also requires appropriate facilities and strict timetabling within the student's existing curriculum (Patrício et al, 2009).

What happens on the day of the OSCE?

Exam etiquette

Prior to your OSCE, your university will contact your regarding your allocated date and time of your examination – each student will have an individual start time.

You should aim to arrive 10 minutes before your first station. If you are late, most universities will not permit you to sit the OSCE at your allocated time and your circumstances will be reviewed on an individual basis. It is your responsibility to check that you attend the OSCE assessment on the correct date and at the correct time. You are unlikely to be permitted to swap your assessment slot without discussing this with the OSCE Lead for your university.

Most universities will require that you dress professionally, which includes adhering to the dress code specified during the clinical placements as listed in the following.

Dress code

- Male students should wear trousers and a shirt. If female students wear a skirt or dress, it should be knee length or below. Trainers, jeans or showing your midriff are not acceptable. Consider how you expect a professional to dress and aspire to a similar standard.

- The sleeves of your shirt, cardigan or top should not be below your elbow; if sleeves are longer, they can be rolled up to this point.
- Male students who wear a tie will need to tuck it between the 3rd and 4th button of their shirt whilst in clinical areas.
- Students with long hair are expected to tie it back.
- In relation to jewellery – watches, bracelets and rings containing stones are not permitted, just plain wedding bands and simple stud earrings. Nail varnish or false nails should not be worn.

You must bring a pen with you, but all other materials will be provided.

Upon entering the exam room

For most pharmacy OSCEs, OSCE stations are either verbal or written and are time limited. The time limit will vary according to your university, but it is usually between 5 and 20 minutes per station. The number of OSCE stations will vary from university to university, however you will be informed of these details prior to the assessment day.

Verbal stations

If it is a verbal station, you will have a specified time to complete the scenario (this includes preparation and performing time). At verbal stations, there will be one or two people present: the patient/doctor/nurse with whom you need to interact and also an examiner who will observe the interaction and mark the OSCE. In some universities, the examiner will also play the standardised patient or doctor.

Written stations

As with verbal stations, you will have a specified time to prepare and complete the scenario. At the written station, nobody will be present. The OSCE coordinator may ask you to place your completed answer sheet into a box beside your OSCE table before you leave the OSCE station.

Content of OSCEs and resources provided

All of the OSCEs are based on information that you have been taught during your course to date, including workshops and placements. You will not be expected to describe the pharmacology of drugs, management plans or mechanisms of drug interactions in great detail but you are expected to have a good overall understanding of the management of common conditions and be able to apply your knowledge to patient management.

At the OSCE station

You will encounter:
1. A table with a copy of the task
2. Verbal station:
   - A SP or healthcare professional (HCP) for you to interact with and an examiner
3. Written station:
   - A written task to be completed
4. Any necessary equipment for the station e.g. an insulin pen, a Peak Expiratory Flow Rate (PEFR) meter, an inhaler, medication kardex, discharge prescription, patient notes

5. Reference sources
6. An answer sheet or notes page

The key to interacting with the 'patients' or 'HCPs' at the verbal OSCE station is to relate to them exactly as you would with real-life patients or healthcare professionals.

You are expected to communicate in an empathetic manner and answer any questions that they might have.

You are responsible for your own time management during the OSCE but an examiner will inform you when you have 2 minutes left and also when the allocated time is completed and it is time to move to the next station. Should you finish early, you may choose to add or change your response. You are to remain at the OSCE station and not engage the patient/ HCP or examiner in conversation.

Marking of OSCEs

Your final mark is based on a standardised marking scheme. The standardised marking scheme is designed so you receive a mark for successfully performing the task related to the item on the checklist. Some items are considered to be multi-factorial and will therefore receive a higher weighting.

Your university may include 'essential' criteria which must be included in the student's answer in order to pass the OSCE. This generally relates to a patient safety issue, which could place patient care at risk if not addressed. If the students do not identify this 'essential' criterion, they will FAIL the OSCE.

Your university may also include a section in their marking scheme to reflect the situation where a student provides information to the patient/doctor which is considered unsafe or breaches legal requirements. This will usually result in a further loss of marks i.e. up to 100% of the total mark available. Not all incidents can be predicted on sample checklists and marking schemes. If an incident occurs in which the OSCE may be failed this will be discussed with another examiner. Examples of some OSCEs and their marking schemes are included in this booklet.

Table 1.1 An example of a professionalism and communication skills scale used during OSCE	
Professionalism including communication style	
Excellent	**All of the time:** appropriately attentive with patient; empathetic and interested; identifies and resolves problems e.g. if patient drinks or smokes, attempted health promotion; doesn't cause embarrassment or loss of face to patient; checks patient understanding by asking repeating back (history taking), organised questioning / provision of information; body language appropriate & eye contact good. **4**
Good	**Most of the time** (as above) **3**
Average	**Some of the time** (as above) **2**
Poor	**Most of the time:** inattentive with patient; lack of empathy and interest; lack of problem identification or resolution; causes embarrassment or loss of face to patient; omitted check of patient understanding by repeating back (history taking), disorganised questioning / provision of information; body language inappropriate & eye contact poor. **1**
Fail	**All of the time** (as above) **0**

Communication skills

During the verbal OSCE stations, you are assessed not only on your knowledge but also on your professionalism and communication style. Table 1.1 gives you an idea of how this may be assessed by the examiner.

Further reading

Adamo, G., 2003. Simulated and standardised patients in OSCEs: achievements and challenges 1992–2003. Med. Teach. 25 (3), 262–270.

Arnold, R.C., Walmsley, A.D., 2008. The use of the OSCE in postgraduate education. Eur. J. Dent. Educ. 12, 126–130.

Austin, Z., Gregory, P., Tabak, D., 2006. Simulated patients versus standardized patients in Objective Structured Clinical Examination. Am. J. Pharm. Educ. 70 (5), Article 119.

Awaisu, A., Abd Rahman, N.S., Nik Mohamed, M.H., et al., 2010. Malaysian Pharmacy Students' Assessment of an Objective Structured Clinical Examination (OSCE). Am. J. Pharm. Educ. 74 (2), Article 34.

Awaisu, A., Mohamed, M.H.N., Mohammad, Q.A., 2007. Perception of Pharmacy Students in Malaysia on the Use of Objective Structured Clinical Examinations to Evaluate Competence. Am. J. Pharm. Educ. 71 (6), Article 118.

Barrows, H.S., Abrahamson, S., 1964. The programmed patient: a technique for appraising student performance in clinical neurology. J. Med. Educ. 39 (8), 802–805.

Beck, D.E., Boh, L.E., O'Sullivan, P.S., 1995. Evaluation of student performance in experiential settings with confidence. Am. J. Pharm. Educ. 59, 236–247.

Corbo, M., Patel, J.P., Abdel Tawab, R., Davies, J.G., 2006. Evaluating clinical skills of undergraduate pharmacy students using objective structured clinical examinations (OSCEs). Pharm. Educ. 6 (1), 5–58.

Crossley, J., Humphries, G., Jolly, B., 2002. Assessing Health Professionals. Med. Educ. 36, 800–804.

Department of Health (DOH), 2006. The Regulation of Non-Medical Healthcare Professions (The Foster Review). The Stationary Office, London, H.M.S.O.

Department of Health (DOH), 2007. Report of the Working Party on Professional Regulation and Leadership in Pharmacy. The Stationary Office, London, H.M.S.O. (DOH, 2007a) (The Clarke Inquiry).

Department of Health (DOH), 2007. Trust, Assurance and Safety. The regulation of Health Professionals in the 21st Century. The Stationary Office, London, H.M.S.O. (DOH, 2007b).

Dupras, D.M., Li, J.T.C., 1995. Use of an objective structured clinical examination to determine clinical competence. Acad. Med. 70, 1029–1034.

Evans, B.W., Alinier, G., Kostrzewski, A.J., et al., 2011. Development and design of Objective Structured Clinical Examination (OSCE) in undergraduate education in a new School of Pharmacy in England. Curr. Pharm. Teach. Learn. 3 (3), 216–223.

Evans, B.W., Kravitz, L., Walker, N., 2013. Pharmacy OSCEs: A Revision Guide. The Pharmaceutical Press, London-Chicago.

Gallimore, C., George, A.K., Brown, M.C., 2008. Pharmacy Students' Preferences for Various Types of Simulated Patients. Am. J. Pharm. Educ. 72 (1), article 01.

General Pharmaceutical Council, 2011. Initial Standards for the Education and Training of Pharmacists. [online] Available at: <http://www.pharmacyregulation.org/regulatingpharmacy/standardsandquality/initialeducation andtrainingforpharmacists/index.aspx> (accessed on 25.05.16).

Harden, R.M., 1990. Twelve tips for organizing an objective structured clinical examination (OSCE). Med. Teach. 12, 259–264.

Harden, R.M., Stevenson, M., Downne, W.W., Wilson, G.M., 1975. Assessment of clinical competence using an observed structured clinical examination (OSCE). Br. Med. J. 1, 447–451.

Hastings, J.K., Flowers, S.K., Pace, A.C., Spadaro, D., 2010. An Objective Standardized Clinical Examination (OSCE) in an Advanced Nonprescription Medicines Course. Am. J. Pharm. Educ. 74 (6), Article 98.

Hodden, R.V., Rivington, R.N., Calcutt, L.E., Haut, I.R., 1989. The effectiveness of immediate feedback during objective structured clinical examination (OSCE). Med. Educ. 23, 184–188.

Hodges, B., 2003. Validity and the OSCE. Med. Teach. 25 (3), 250–254. Hodges, 2003a.

Hughes, F., Barry, J., Belaid, L., et al., 2013. Development of an Objective Structured Clinical Examination (OSCE) to assess formulation and extemporaneous dispensing skills in MPharm undergraduates. Pharmacy Education 13 (1), 7–14.

Jeffries, A., Simmons, B., Tabak, D., et al., 2007. Using an objective structured clinical examination (OSCE) to assess multiple physician competencies in postgraduate training. Med. Teach. 29, 183–191.

Langford, N.J., Landray, M., Kendall, M.J., Ferner, R.E., 2004. Testing the practical aspects of therapeutics by objective structured clinical examination. J. Clin. Pharm. Ther. 29, 263–266.

Mavis, B.E., 2000. Does studying for an objective structured clinical examination make a difference? Med. Educ. 34, 808–812.

Patrício, M., Miguel, J., Fareleira, F., et al., 2009. A comprehensive checklist for reporting the use of OSCEs. Med. Teach. 31, 112–124.

Quero Munoz, L., O'Byrne, C., Pugsley, J., Austin, Z., 2005. Reliability, validity and generalisability of an objective structured clinical examination (OSCE) for assessment of entry-to-practice in pharmacy. Pharmacy Education 5 (1), 33–43.

Ragan, R.E., Virtue, D.W., Chi, S.J., 2013. An Assessment Program Using Standardised Clients to Determine Student Readiness for Clinical Practice. Am. J. Pharm. Educ. 77 (1), article 14.

Ragucci, K.R., Fermo, J.D., Mazur, J.N., 2005. Objective structured clinical examinations for an ambulatory care pharmacy rotation. Am. J. Health Syst. Pharm. 62, 927–929.

Royal Pharmaceutical Society of Great Britain (RPSGB), 1996. The New Horizon: Pharmacy in a New Age. The Royal Pharmaceutical Society of Great Britain, London.

Royal Pharmaceutical Society of Great Britain (RPSGB), 2004. Making Pharmacy Education Fit for the Future. Available at <http://www.rpsgb.org.uk/pdfs/maphedfitforfuturesumm.pdf> (accessed on 25.05.16).

Salinitri, F.D., O'Connell, M.B., Garwood, C.L., et al., 2012. An Objective Structured Clinical Examination to Assess Problem-Based Learning. Am. J. Pharm. Educ. 76 (3), Article 44.

Schoonheim-Klein, M.E., Habets, L.L.M.H., Aartman, I.H.A., et al., 2006. Implementing an objective structured clinical examination (OSCE) in dental education: effects on students' learning strategies. Eur. J. Dent. Educ. 10, 226–235.

Schultz, K.W., Kirby, J., Delva, D., et al., 2004. Medical students and residents preferred site characteristic and preceptor behaviours for learning in the ambulatory setting: a cross-sectional survey. BMC Med. Educ. 4 (12).

Schwartzman, E., Hus, D.I., Law, A.V., Chung, E.P., 2011. Assessment of patient counseling skills during objective structured clinical examination: examining the effectiveness of a training program in minimising inter-grader variability. Patient Educ. Couns. 83, 472–477.

Shumway, J.M., Harden, R.M., 2003. AMEE Guide No. 25: the assessment of learning for the competent and reflective physician. Med. Teach. 25 (6), 569–584.

Smith, D., 2002. Not by Error but by Design – Harold Shipman and the Regulatory Crisis for Health Care. Public Policy Adm. 17 (4), 55–74.

Sturpe, D., 2010. Objective Structured Clinical Examinations in Doctor of Pharmacy Programs in the United States. Am. J. Pharm. Educ. 74 (8), Article 148.

Swanson, D.B., Norcini, J.J., 1989. Factors influencing reliability of tests using standardised patients. Teach. Learn. Med. 1, 158–166.

Tamblyn, R.M., Klass, D.V., Schabl, G.K., Kopelow, M.L., 1991. Sources of unreliability and bias in standardised patient rating. Teach. Learn. Med. 3, 74–85.

The Elizabeth Lee case. Available at <http://www.pharmaceutical-journal.com/news-and-analysis/former-locum-handed-suspended-jail-term-for-dispensing-error/10882780.article> (accessed on 25.05.16).

The Mid-Staffordshire Public Inquiry. Available at <http://webarchive.nationalarchives.gov.uk/20150407084003/http://www.midstaffspublicinquiry.com/report> (Accessed on 25.05.16).

Turner, J.L., Dankoski, M.E., 2008. Objective Structured Clinical Exams: A critical review. Fam. Med. 40 (8), 574–578.

van der Vleuten, C.P.M., Swanson, D.B., 1990. Assessment of clinical skills with standardized patients: state of the art. Teach. Learn. Med. 2 (2), 58–76.

9

Dispensed medication

When dealing with dispensed medication, one of the key skills of a pharmacist is to perform a *clinical assessment* or *clinical check* of the medicine to be supplied.

Clinical checks involve identifying potential problems by collecting and assessing all of the information that you have available on the patient and his or her medication. In order to perform a clinical check correctly you must consider all that you know about the patient and the medicine. This includes thinking about the patient's disease state, how the medicines prescribed actually work and how all of these aspects of care will come together.

When completing a clinical check it is best to have a systematic approach (Box 2.1). In your MPharm course you may have developed your own standard operating procedure (SOP) for performing this task. Use your own standard operating procedure (SOP) to approach the stations or look at the information below to help you to develop a process.

Box 2.1

How to... complete an accuracy check and a clinical and legal check on a community prescription (adapted from NPA SOP guidance)

Accuracy check

This can be carried out by a qualified accuracy checking technician (ACT) or pharmacist

- Read whole prescription
- Check each item individually in the order that they appear on the prescription
- Cross check the label(s) and medicinal product(s) against the prescription for:
  - Name of medicine
  - Strength of the product
  - Formulation of the product
  - Quantity of the product
- Check the label(s) against the prescription for:
  - Name of patient
  - Dosage instructions

Continued

Box 2.1—Cont'd

- Also check that:
  - A patient information leaflet (PIL) is included for each medicinal product
  - For medicines which were dispensed from bulk packs check that the contents of the stock pack match the contents of the dispensed medicinal product
  - Check expiry date on each product
  - Appropriate BNF warnings appear on label
- For oral liquid formulations add an appropriate plastic spoon or oral syringe

Clinical and legal check

This should be carried out by the pharmacist only

- Check that prescription complies with all legal requirements. Take particular care with controlled drug prescriptions
- Take into account the following factors where thought to be significant and assess the prescription for clinical appropriateness:
  - Age of patient
  - Sex of patient
  - Weight of patient
  - Pregnant or breastfeeding
  - Relevant clinical condition
  - Interactions
  - Dose
  - Formulation
  - Cautions and contraindications
  - Allergies
- Where the prescription may not be clinically appropriate take steps to obtain additional information in order to come to a final decision. Consider:
  - Discussing issues with prescriber
  - Discussing issues with patient
  - Checking appropriate reference sources
- Where the prescription is legally valid and clinically appropriate then prepare any notes you wish to discuss

Look at the patient first:

- *Patient characteristics.* Do they belong to a specialist group e.g. elderly, pregnant or breastfeeding women, children? Ethnicity may also have an influence on some doses of medication. Gender will have an effect on some medications e.g. finasteride is contraindicated for women.
- *What are the other co-morbidities?* E.g. does the patient suffer from renal or hepatic impairment? Do you have access to this clinical information?

- *Patient preferences.* E.g. this may be related to previous experiences with different formulations or religious beliefs and certain formulations.
- *Allergies.* E.g. active ingredients and excipients.

Look at the medicine:

- *Indication.* E.g. has the patient been diagnosed with a new set of symptoms or disease state? Is it a new medicine for an existing indication? Has another medicine been discontinued?
- *Dose, frequency & strength.* Check if these are appropriate and safe for the individual patient. Double check paediatric doses where possible.
- *Dosing of the formulation.* Check that the prescribed dosing is appropriate for the formulation.
- *Interactions and drug compatibility.* Is the patient on other medicines that may be affected or contraindicated?
- *Monitoring requirements.* E.g. if the patient is on warfarin, what was their last international normalized ratio (INR)?
- *Route.* E.g. check issues relating to route.
- *Administration aids.* Check the need for adherence aids e.g. oral syringe in an appropriate size, spacers, eye drop devices, verbal information.

How to... clinically screen for medications on a hospital inpatient's medication kardex

Reviewing or clinically screening medications should be done in a *stepwise* fashion to ensure each medication is safe and suitable for each individual patient. Keep patient safety forefront in all of your decision making.

There isn't always a clear cut solution, and your clinical judgement should always be used. When a number of options exist, they may need to be weighed up on a risk-benefit basis so as to decide on the most appropriate plan of action.

We outline here a stepwise approach to clinically screening inpatient medication prescriptions – in this case, a medication kardex (see Fig. 2.1).

Look at the patient first:

- *Patient characteristics.* Do they belong to a specialist group e.g. elderly, pregnant or breastfeeding women, children? Ethnicity may have an influence on risk factors e.g. in coronary heart disease, diabetes.
- *What are the other co-morbidities?* E.g. does the patient suffer from renal or hepatic impairment? Does a co-morbid state affect drug choice in the management of acute admission? E.g. is the patient asthmatic and require a beta-blocker? Whilst this combination is used regularly, the patient must be informed of the risk of impact on asthmatic management.
- *Patient preferences.* E.g. a patient with atrial fibrillation as a new diagnosis who requires thromboprophylaxis – they have a choice of warfarin or any of the direct oral anticoagulants. The options, pros and cons of each treatment must be explained in patient friendly terms so the patient can come to the best decision about his or her own healthcare.
- *Allergies.* E.g. active ingredients and excipients, classes of drugs.

13

Look at the medicine:

- *Indication.* E.g. is there an indication for each medication, why is it prescribed? Is it contra-indicated in this patient or in this condition? Is there therapeutic duplication?
- *Trigger or high risk drug?* Is the medication considered a high risk drug e.g. due to a narrow therapeutic index (digoxin, warfarin), high risk of adverse effects (methotrexate, gentamicin) or interactions (simvastatin, clarithromycin).
- *Dose, frequency & strength.* Check if these are appropriate and safe for the individual patient. Double check doses in extremes of age; elderly and neonate / paediatric, check patient weight for all paediatric and neonate and note the DATE the weight is recorded for all neonates.
- *Dosing of the formulation.* Check the prescribed dosing is appropriate for the formulation and that the prescribing formulation is the most appropriate for the patient.
- *Interactions and drug compatibility.* Is the patient on other medicines that may be affected or contraindicated? Is the patient aware of the interactions with food / alcohol or co-morbid states? Rivaroxaban **must** be taken with food.
- *Monitoring requirements.* Depending on the medication – consider checking BP, HR, and renal function plus calculating CrCl, checking U&E, FBC, LFTs, antibiotic titres etc.
- *Route.* For example, in a patient who has had a stroke and has dysphagia, all oral medications must be reviewed – can they be given via another route, and if not, what alternatives are suitable for this patient?
- *Administration aids.* Check the need for adherence aids as described previously including the use of a Dosette® or Medi-Dose®, commonly seen as a way of improving patient adherence when pill burdens increase. This is not always the answer and close collaboration with patients regarding their lifestyles and choices should support the decision for compliance aids. There are a number of decision tools available to support this decision.

Figure 2.1 An example of a blank medication kardex used to administer medication in a hospital setting.

Continued

Venous Thromboembolism (VTE) Risk Assessment for Hospitalised Adults

Risk assessment must be completed on admission

Write in CAPITAL LETTERS or use addressograph

Surname: ....

First Names: ....

Hospital No: ....

DOB: .... *Check identity*

Step 1: Assess for level of mobility – All Patients

	Tick		Tick		Tick
Surgical patient		Medical patient expected to have ongoing reduced mobility relative to normal state		Medical patient NOT expected to have significantly reduced mobility relative to normal state	
Assess for thrombosis and bleeding risk below (Complete steps 2 – 5)				Risk assessment complete (Go to step 5)☒	

Step 2: Review thrombosis risk
Any tick for thrombosis risk factors should prompt consideration for thromboprophylaxis

Patient related	Tick	Admission related	Tick
Active cancer or cancer treatment		Significantly reduced mobility for 3 days or more	
Age >60		Hip or knee replacement	
Dehydration		Hip fracture	
Known thrombophilias		Total anaesthetic + surgery time > 90 minutes	
Personal history / first degree relative with history of VTE		Surgery involving pelvis or lower limb with anaesthetic + surgery time > 60 minutes	
One or more significant medical comorbidities (eg heart disease; metabolic, endocrine or respiratory pathologies; acute infectious diseases; inflammatory conditions)		Acute surgical admission with inflammatory or intra-abdominal condition	
Obesity (BMI>30kg/m^2)		Critical care admission	
Use of hormone replacement therapy		Surgery with significant reduction in mobility	
Use of oestrogen-containing oral contraceptive therapy		**The above risk factors are not exhaustive, additional risks may be considered. Other:**	
Varicose veins with phlebitis			
Pregnancy or < 6 weeks post partum (see obstetric risk assessment for VTE)			

Step 3: Review bleeding risk
Any tick should prompt staff to consider if bleeding risk is sufficient to preclude pharmacological intervention

Patient related	Tick	Admission related	Tick
Active bleeding		Neurosurgery, spinal surgery or eye surgery	
Acquired bleeding disorder (such as acute liver failure)		Lumbar puncture / epidural / spinal anaesthesia expected in the next 12 hours	
Concurrent use of anticoagulants known to increase risk of bleeding (such as warfarin with INR >2)		Lumbar puncture / epidural / spinal anaesthesia within the previous 4 hours	
Acute stroke		Other procedure with high bleeding risk	
Thrombocytopaenia (Platelets <75x10^9/l)		**The above risk factors are not exhaustive, additional risks may be considered. Other:**	
Uncontrolled systolic hypertension (>230/120)			
Untreated inherited bleeding disorder (such as haemophilia and von Willebrand's disease)			

Step 4: Tick the appropriate risk category

Risk of VTE (tick)	High risk of VTE with low bleeding risk		High risk of VTE with significant bleeding risk		Low risk of VTE	
Thromboprophylaxis prescribed on kardex? (tick)	Yes		Type Prescribed (tick)	Pharmacological e.g. LMWH		
	No			Mechanical		

Step 5: Signature

VTE risk assessed on admission	Signature:	Print Name:	Date and Time:

VTE risk should be re-assessed within 24 hours and whenever clinical condition changes

Northern Ireland VTE Advisory Group, June 2011

Figure 2.1—cont'd

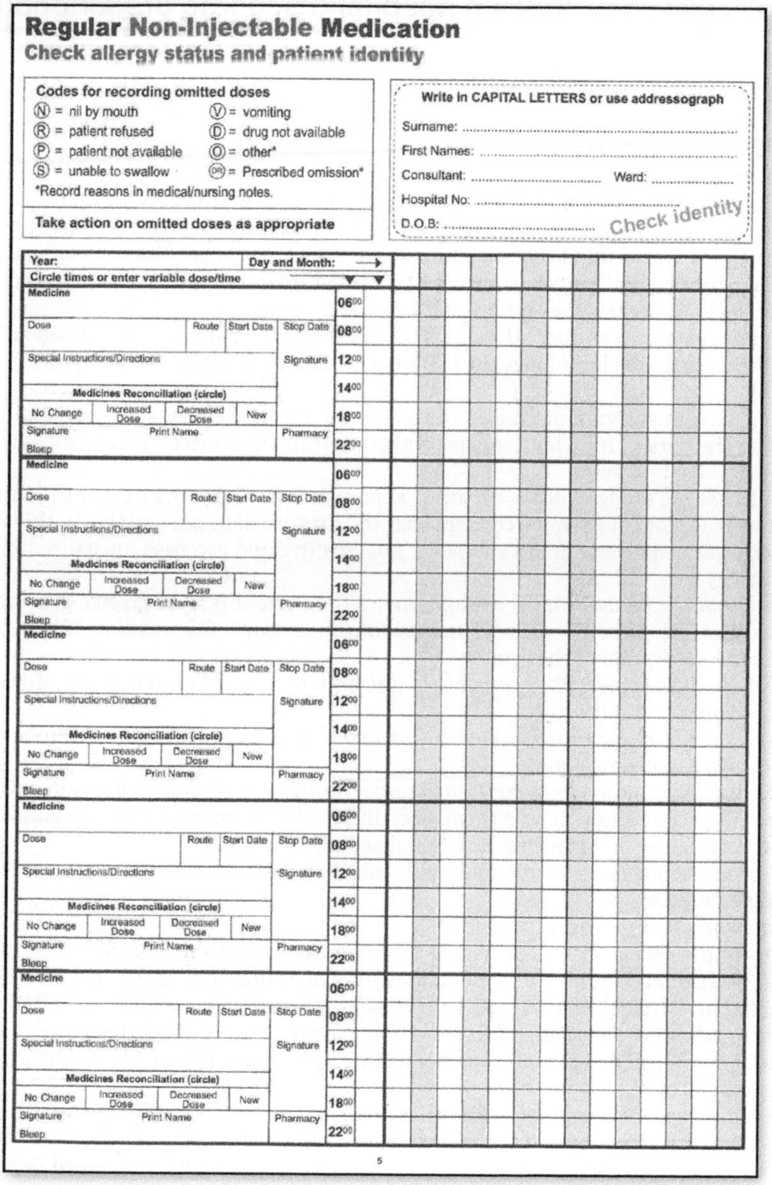

Regular Non-Injectable Medication

Check allergy status and patient identity

Codes for recording omitted doses

Ⓝ = nil by mouth
Ⓡ = patient refused
Ⓟ = patient not available
Ⓢ = unable to swallow
Ⓥ = vomiting
Ⓓ = drug not available
Ⓞ = other*
(OR) = Prescribed omission*

*Record reasons in medical/nursing notes.

Take action on omitted doses as appropriate

Write in CAPITAL LETTERS or use addressograph

Surname: ....

First Names: ....

Consultant: .... Ward: ....

Hospital No: ....

D.O.B: .... Check identity

Year: | **Day and Month:** →

Circle times or enter variable dose/time

Medicine
Dose | Route | Start Date | Stop Date
Special Instructions/Directions | Signature
Medicines Reconciliation (circle)
No Change | Increased Dose | Decreased Dose | New
Signature | Print Name | Pharmacy
Bleep
06:00, 08:00, 12:00, 14:00, 18:00, 22:00

Medicine
Dose | Route | Start Date | Stop Date
Special Instructions/Directions | Signature
Medicines Reconciliation (circle)
No Change | Increased Dose | Decreased Dose | New
Signature | Print Name | Pharmacy
Bleep
06:00, 08:00, 12:00, 14:00, 18:00, 22:00

Medicine
Dose | Route | Start Date | Stop Date
Special Instructions/Directions | Signature
Medicines Reconciliation (circle)
No Change | Increased Dose | Decreased Dose | New
Signature | Print Name | Pharmacy
Bleep
06:00, 08:00, 12:00, 14:00, 18:00, 22:00

Medicine
Dose | Route | Start Date | Stop Date
Special Instructions/Directions | Signature
Medicines Reconciliation (circle)
No Change | Increased Dose | Decreased Dose | New
Signature | Print Name | Pharmacy
Bleep
06:00, 08:00, 12:00, 14:00, 18:00, 22:00

Medicine
Dose | Route | Start Date | Stop Date
Special Instructions/Directions | Signature
Medicines Reconciliation (circle)
No Change | Increased Dose | Decreased Dose | New
Signature | Print Name | Pharmacy
Bleep
06:00, 08:00, 12:00, 14:00, 18:00, 22:00

5

Figure 2.1—cont'd

How to... clinically check a hospital discharge prescription

Suggested stepwise approach to clinically screening inpatient medications:

1. *Check the age of the patient.* If the prescription is for a child check the weight; with a neonate, note the weight and the date of weighing. Check if they require liquid or suspension formulations.

2. *Check the ward the patient has come from.* If it is a maternity ward, is the patient pregnant or breastfeeding? What impact does this have on the prescription?

3. *Check the reason for admission.* Ensure that the medications prescribed are safe and effective bearing in mind the reason for admission. Are any medications omitted? E.g., if admitted with an ST elevation Myocardial Infarction (STEMI) and no statin is prescribed – is there a reason for this?

4. *Check the patient's co-morbid states.* For example if the patient is prescribed an antidepressant which prolongs the QT interval in a patient with an arrhythmia, is this safe?

5. *Check each medication* prescribed to ensure the dose and frequency is suitable and safe for the patient for whom it is prescribed bearing in mind the patient's co-morbid states.

6. *Check that the dosage form* is the most appropriate for the patient e.g. if the patient has a short bowel or colostomy – confirm that the formulations are suitable in this case, some sustained release preparations are not effective and can pass unchanged into the colostomy bag.

7. *Check that the dosage form is appropriate for the route* it is to be given e.g. if the medication has to be given via a Percutaneous Endoscopic Gastrostomy (PEG) does this affect the absorption of the drug?

8. *Are all medicines prescribed generically* (except where brand prescribing is indicated e.g. theophylline preparations)?

9. *Do all short-term medications have a stop date stated* e.g. antibiotics, electrolyte supplements, prednisolone?

10. *Have any medications been continued unnecessarily* e.g. sleeping tablets in patients who only receive these to help them sleep in hospital, nebules in patients admitted with acute respiratory problems but now stabilised on inhalers etc.

11. *Are there any medications missing* e.g. breakthrough pain relief in a patient receiving a modified release opioid?

12. *Is there any therapeutic duplication?*

13. *Is any of the therapy contra-indicated* based on the patient's diagnosis?

14. *Is all medication required to treat the diagnosis prescribed* e.g. anticoagulants for atrial fibrillation, Glyceryl Trinitrate (GTN) spray in Ischaemic Heart Disease (IHD)?

15. *Is the medication considered 'high risk' or a 'trigger' drug* i.e. requiring more thorough consideration e.g. due to a narrow therapeutic index, high risk of adverse effects or interactions etc?

16. *Does the medication interact* with other medications / disease state / food?

17. *Is the patient allergic* to any of the medicines prescribed?

18. *Check discharge prescription* for legalities e.g. ensure prescription is signed (legal requirement).

An example discharge is displayed below.

The Hospital

| DISCHARGE AND MEDICATION ADVICE LETTER |

DR NAME + ADDRESS

GP CODE:

Patient Name
Patient Address

Admission Date:	**30/06/2016**	Phone No:	**02890666666**
Admission Method:	**Via A&E**	DOB:	Age:
Discharge Date:		Sex:	**M/F** (delete as applicable)
Discharge Method:	**Discharge to home**	H&C No:	353 684 8960
Ward:	**Ward One**		
Discharging Consultant:	**Dr Name**		

CURRENT EPISODE DETAILS

Principal Diagnosis:	
Underlying Conditions & Co-Morbidities:	
Procedures/Dates:	
Relevant clinical concerns:	

FOLLOW UP PLANS	COMMENTS
Outstanding Investigations:	
Hospital Review Arrangements:	
Additional Care Arrangements:	
Action Required By GP:	

Figure 2.2 An example of a Discharge and Medication advice letter that the hospital will send to the GP on a patient discharge from hospital.

Continued

Example 2.1. OSCE Station: Accuracy and clinical check for a community prescription

Please read the following information carefully. You have 10 minutes to complete the task.

Background

Your dispenser has dispensed a prescription for Mrs Aoife Kavanagh (68 years old).

Medical history

Mrs Kavanagh suffers from hypercholesterolaemia (raised cholesterol) which is being successfully managed with a statin (simvastatin).
The patient has presented to your community pharmacy with a prescription which contains a new medication for a fungal infection known as tinea corporis (ringworm).

Task

1. Review Mrs Kavanagh's prescription and dispensed items.
2. Identify any **accuracy, legal or clinical issues** with the dispensed prescription.
3. Where issues are identified, document these on the answer sheet provided with the required actions.

Please do NOT write on or remove materials provided.

Please submit your answer sheet to the examiner at the end of the OSCE, and do not forget to include your name

Station props that would be provided

Item required:

1. Instructions for candidate.

2. Copy of instructions for examiner.

3. Candidate answer sheet.

4. Mark Sheet.

5. BNF.

6. Labels

7. Community prescription.

8. Stockley – https://www.medicinescomplete.com/mc/stockley/2010/

Labels for prescription (for OSCE 2.1)

Keep out of the reach and sight of children.

14 Sporanox® 100 mg capsules.
Take TWO capsules DAILY for 7 days.
Do not take indigestion remedies 2 hours before or after you take this medicine. Space the doses evenly throughout the day. Keep taking this medicine until the course is finished unless you are told to stop.
Take with or just after food, or a meal.
Swallow this medicine whole. Do not chew or crush.
Aoife Kavanagh
Today's date   Name of pharmacy and address

Keep out of the reach and sight of children

28 Simvastatin 20 mg Tablets
Take ONE as directed

Aoife Kavanagh
Today's date   Name of pharmacy and address

NHS Prescription from a General Practitioner

Rev 01/14 Pharmacy stamp and date *Pharmacy stamp*	Age **68 years** DOB	Name (including forename) and address **Mrs Aoife Kavanagh** **1 Hudson Heights** **Irvinestown**
No. of days treatment	NHS No.	Code numbers

Sporanox capsules

200 mg daily for 7 days

Simvastatin 20 mg tablets

20 mg nocte

×28

Signature of Prescriber Prescriber's normal signature	Date Today's date

Prescriber's Details

All correct

| PATIENTS – please read the notes overleaf | | Form Number |

Figure 2.3 Mrs Kavanagh's prescription form (for OSCE 2.1).

OSCE Answer sheet (for OSCE 2.1)

Candidate name:		Date:	
Issue:		**Action(s) needed:**	

NHS Prescription from a General Practitioner

Rev 01/14 Pharmacy stamp and date *Pharmacy stamp*	Age **59 years** DOB	Name (including forename) and address **James Burtin** **49 Fairview Park** **Aberdeen**

No. of days treatment		NHS No.		Code numbers

Camcolit 400 mg MR tablets

400 mg BD

×100

Diclofenac sodium 75 mg MR tablets

75 mg BD

×14

Signature of Prescriber Prescriber's signature	Date Today's date

Prescriber's Details

All correct

PATIENTS – please read the notes overleaf | | Form Number

Figure 2.4 Mr Burtin's prescription form (for OSCE 2.2).

OSCE Answer sheet (for OSCE 2.2)	
Candidate name:	Date:
Issue:	Action(s) needed:

Example 2.3. OSCE Station

Please read the following information carefully. You have 10 minutes to complete the task.

Background

You are working as a community pharmacist and have been asked to undertake a final accuracy and clinical check on the NHS prescription for Joseph Subair. The prescription has been dispensed by the dispensing assistant in the pharmacy.

The parent of Joseph who is waiting to collect the medicines confirms that he has no allergies and weighs 19.2 kg. Joseph has been started on a new treatment (Epanutin®) in order to treat focal seizures.

Task

1. Review Joseph Subair's prescription and dispensed items.
2. Identify any accuracy, legal or clinical issues with the dispensed prescription.
3. Where issues are identified, document these on the answer sheet provided with the required actions.

Please submit your completed answer sheet to the examiner at the end of the OSCE, and do not forget to include your name.

Please do not write on any of the provided resources.

Station props that would be provided

Item required:

1. Instructions for candidate.

2. Copy of instructions for examiner.

3. Candidate answer sheet.

4. Mark Sheet.

5. BNF.

6. Labels.

7. Community prescription.

Labels for prescription (for OSCE 2.3)

Keep out of the reach and sight of children

500 mL Epanutin Suspension 30 mg/5 mL
Give 6 mL using the oral syringe provided TWICE daily
Shake the bottle
Warning: Do not stop taking this medicine unless your doctor tells you to stop.

Joseph Subair
Today's date   Name of pharmacy and address

Keep out of reach and sight of children

500 mL Doublebase emollient bath additive
Apply liberally as directed

Joseph Subair
Today's date   Name of pharmacy and address

NHS Prescription from a General Practitioner

Rev 01/14	Age	Name (including forename) and address
Pharmacy stamp and date *Pharmacy stamp*	5 years DOB 2 months	Joseph Subair 49 Main Street Banbridge

No. of days treatment		NHS No.		Code numbers

Epanutin Suspension 30 mg / 5 mL

48 mg BD

×500 mL

Doublebase Dayleve Gel 15%

Apply liberally as directed

×500 g

Signature of Prescriber	Date
Prescriber's signature	Today's date

Prescriber's Details

All correct

PATIENTS – please read the notes overleaf

Form Number

Figure 2.5 Mr Subair's prescription (for OSCE 2.3).

OSCE Answer sheet (for OSCE 2.3)

Candidate name:		Date:	
Issue:		**Action(s) needed:**	

Example 2.4. OSCE: Clinical Check of a hospital discharge prescription

Please read the following information carefully. You have 10 minutes to complete the task.

Background

You are working in the dispensary as a pharmacist, performing clinical checks on **discharge prescriptions**.

You receive a discharge prescription from the Medical Assessment Unit, written by the F1 doctor, for Mr Seamus McKenna who presented with a painful inflamed knee and has been prescribed analgesia.

Task

Complete all aspects of the **answer sheet** provided to:

1. **Clinically check** Mr Seamus McKenna's discharge prescription (i.e. review the prescription to ensure the *safety and efficacy* of the medicines prescribed and assess the *accuracy and legality* of the prescription).

2. **Document** any **safety, legal** or **accuracy** issues you identify which require resolution and **indicate how you would resolve these.**

Please submit your completed answer to the examiner at the end of the OSCE and do not forget to include your name on the form.

DO NOT write on or remove any materials provided.

Station props that would be provided

Item required:

1. Candidate answer sheet.

2. Mark Sheet.

3. BNF

4. Mr Seamus McKenna's medication kardex (see Fig. 2.6)

5. Mr Seamus McKenna's discharge prescription (see Fig. 2.7)

WQA7000 Rev. October 2011

Medicine Prescription and Administration Record

Rewritten on (date): x/xx/xx
Record: 1 of 1

Allergies / Medicine Sensitivities

THIS SECTION MUST BE COMPLETED

Date	Medicine (generic) / Allergen	Type of Reaction	Signature

OR

No Known allergies ✓ Please tick

Signature: _F.Rover_   Date: x/xx/xx

Write in CAPITAL LETTERS or use addressograph

Surname: McKenna
First Names: Seamus
Hospital No: 123456
DOB: 22/11/53

Check identity

Hospital: The Trust   Ward: Ward One
Consultant: Burton
Date of Admission: x/xx/xx

Weight (Kg)	Date	Height (cm)

Admissions Medicines Reconciliation completed

Sign: J. Anderson   Date: x/xx/xx

Discharge prescription ordered by

Sign: F. Rover   Date: x/xx/xx

Requirements for Prescribing and Administration

- Nurses must not administer medicines that are improperly or illegibly prescribed.
- Do not prescribe or administer medication if the allergy status is not documented and signed (unless in an emergency).
- Prescribe generically (refer to WHSCT Policy for appropriate use of approved/generic names of medicines).
- Print the full name of the medicine in CAPITALS in black ink. Do not abbreviate medicine names.
- Do not alter existing instructions. Cancel and rewrite any changes in medicine therapy.
- Discontinue any therapy by drawing a diagonal line through the prescription and the remainder of the administration record. Enter the date of discontinuation and signature in the 'Stop' space.
- Do not abbreviate 'micrograms', 'nanograms', 'international units' or units; write in full.
- Prescriber's signatures must be written in full; initials are not acceptable.
- Other prescriptions in use must be referenced on the main prescription record.
- Attach all additional charts to the Medicine Prescription and Administration record.
- The administering nurse(s) must initial each administration.
- All kardexes must be rewritten after 14 days.
- Medicines reconciliation - for each regular or when required medicine, indicate changes made to therapy during stay.
  - On admission, refer to the patient's documented medication history, reconcile medicines on the kardex and circle 'no change', 'increased dose', 'decreased dose' or 'new' medicine accordingly.
  - During patient stay, ensure any subsequent changes are similarly indicated and document the reason in the table below.
  - At discharge, ensure information on medicine changes (including stopped medication) is sent to the GP.

Additional Charts in Use (please tick)

Epidural ☐	Intrathecal ☐	Blood Sugar Monitoring ☐
Patient Controlled Analgesia ☐	Diabetic Ketoacidosis ☐	Fluid Balance ☐
Insulin ☐	Chemotherapy ☐	Anaesthetic Record ☐

Total Parenteral Nutrition (TPN) ☐	Other (please specify) ☐
Oral Anticoagulant ✓	Syringe Driver (please indicate 1 or more) ☐
Endoscopy ☐	

Special Instructions / Additional Notes on Medicines / Reason for Medicine Omission (please sign and date)

Medicines Reconciliation Record During Patient's Stay

	Medication	Commenced in Hospital (tick if YES)	Stopped in Hospital (tick if YES)	Dose Changed ↑ or ↓	Reason for Medication Change
1					
2					
3					
4					
5					

1

OS17629

Figure 2.6 Mr Seamus McKenna's medication kardex (for OSCE 2.4)

Continued

Regular Non-Injectable Medication
Check allergy status and patient identity

Codes for recording omitted doses

(N) = nil by mouth   (V) = vomiting
(R) = patient refused   (D) = drug not available
(P) = patient not available   (O) = other*
(S) = unable to swallow   (PO) = Prescribed omission*
*Record reasons in medical/nursing notes.

Take action on omitted doses as appropriate

Write in CAPITAL LETTERS or use addressograph

Surname: McKenna
First Names: Seamus
Consultant: Burton   Ward: One
Hospital No: 123456
D.O.B: 22/11/53   *Check identity*

Year: XXXX			Day and Month: →			x/x	x/x	x/x									
Circle times or enter variable dose/time				▼	▼												
Medicine Warfarin					06⁰⁰												
Dose as per INR	Route 0	Start Date x/x	Stop Date		08⁰⁰												
Special Instructions / Directions * See Chart *				Signature	12⁰⁰												
Medicines Reconciliation (circle)					14⁰⁰												
(No Change)	Increased Dose	Decreased Dose	New		(18⁰⁰)	PI	SV	SP									
Signature *FR* Bleep 1234	Print Name F Porter		Pharmacy SP		22⁰⁰												
Medicine Bisoprolol					(06⁰⁰)	MT	SP	SS									
Dose 10 mg	Route 0	Start Date x/x	Stop Date		08⁰⁰												
Special Instructions / Directions				Signature	12⁰⁰												
Medicines Reconciliation (circle)					14⁰⁰												
(No Change)	Increased Dose	Decreased Dose	New		18⁰⁰												
Signature *FR* Bleep 1234	Print Name F Porter		Pharmacy SP		22⁰⁰												
Medicine					06⁰⁰												
Dose	Route	Start Date	Stop Date		08⁰⁰												
Special Instructions / Directions				Signature	12⁰⁰												
Medicines Reconciliation (circle)					14⁰⁰												
No Change	Increased Dose	Decreased Dose	New		18⁰⁰												
Signature Bleep	Print Name		Pharmacy		22⁰⁰												
Medicine					06⁰⁰												
Dose	Route	Start Date	Stop Date		08⁰⁰												
Special Instructions / Directions				Signature	12⁰⁰												
Medicines Reconciliation (circle)					14⁰⁰												
No Change	Increased Dose	Decreased Dose	New		18⁰⁰												
Signature Bleep	Print Name		Pharmacy		22⁰⁰												
Medicine					06⁰⁰												
Dose	Route	Start Date	Stop Date		08⁰⁰												
Special Instructions / Directions				Signature	12⁰⁰												
Medicines Reconciliation (circle)					14⁰⁰												
No Change	Increased Dose	Decreased Dose	New		18⁰⁰												
Signature Bleep	Print Name		Pharmacy		22⁰⁰												

5

Figure 2.6—cont'd

Abbreviations for frequency	Write in CAPITAL LETTERS or use addressograph
Once daily = od Every morning = om or mane Twice daily = bd Every night = on or nocte Three times daily = tds or tid Four times daily = qds or qid	Surname: McKenna First Names: Seamus Hospital Number: 123456 D.O.B: 22/11/53

As Required Medicines
Check for allergies / drug sensitivities

Medicine Paracetamol			Start Date x/xx	Date	x/x	x/x	x/x	x/x										
Dose 1 g	Route 0	Freq. (max) 4-6 hrly	Stop Date	Time	10:00	16:00	22:00	8:00										
Signature F. Porter			Signature	Dose Route	1g 0	1g 0	1g 0	1g 0										
Special Instructions / Directions * 8 daily *			Pharmacy SH	Given by	PP	SM	PM	PP										
Medicine Ibuprofen			Start Date x/xx	Date														
Dose 400 mg	Route 0	Freq. (max) 8 hrly	Stop Date	Time														
Signature F. Porter			Signature	Dose Route														
Special Instructions / Directions			Pharmacy SH	Given by														
Medicine			Start Date	Date														
Dose	Route	Freq. (max)	Stop Date	Time														
Signature			Signature	Dose Route														
Special Instructions / Directions			Pharmacy	Given by														
Medicine			Start Date	Date														
Dose	Route	Freq. (max)	Stop Date	Time														
Signature			Signature	Dose Route														
Special Instructions / Directions			Pharmacy	Given by														
Medicine			Start Date	Date														
Dose	Route	Freq. (max)	Stop Date	Time														
Signature			Signature	Dose Route														
Special Instructions / Directions			Pharmacy	Given by														
Medicine			Start Date	Date														
Dose	Route	Freq. (max)	Stop Date	Time														
Signature			Signature	Dose Route														
Special Instructions / Directions			Pharmacy	Given by														

Omitted Doses of Medication

Date	Time	Medication, Dose and Route	Reason for omission and action taken	Signature

Figure 2.6—cont'd

The Hospital

DISCHARGE AND MEDICATION ADVICE LETTER

DR NAME + ADDRESS
                GP CODE:

Patient Name:	Seamus McKenna
Patient Address:	12th Street

Admission Date:	**30/06/2016**	Phone No:	**02890666666**
Admission Method:	**Via A&E**	DOB:	Age: 63
Discharge Date:		Sex:	(M)/ F (delete as applicable)
Discharge Method:	**Discharge to home**	H&C No:	123456
Ward:	**Ward One**		
Discharging Consultant:	**Dr. Burton**		

CURRENT EPISODE DETAILS

Principal Diagnosis:	Inflamed & painful knee
Underlying Conditions & Co-Morbidities:	Atrial fibrillation
Procedures/Dates:	
Relevant clinical concerns:	Pain control

FOLLOW UP PLANS	COMMENTS
Outstanding Investigations:	N/a
Hospital Review Arrangements:	N/a
Additional Care Arrangements:	N/a
Action Required By GP:	Review pain in 1 week

Figure 2.7   Mr Seamus McKenna's discharge prescription (for OSCE 2.4)

| ALLERGY/DRUG SENSITIVITIES | NKDA | | TYPE OF REACTION (IF KNOWN) | | | |

MEDICATION ON DISCHARGE

Take home supply needed Y/N	MEDICINE (APPROVED NAME)	ROUTE	DOSE AND FREQUENCY	NOTES / COMMENTS DURATION IF APPROPRIATE, INDICATION IF NEW DRUG, TITRATION ETC.	CHANGES N-New I-Increased D-Decreased	PHARMACY INFORMATION (INCLUDING QUANTITY SUPPLIED)
Y	Warfarin	0	3 mg OD	at 6 pm	—	
Y	Bisoprolol	0	10 mg	On going	—	
Y	Ibuprofen	0	400 mg TID	For 3 days	N	

MEDICATION STOPPED	REASON FOR STOPPING

ADDITIONAL MEDICATION INFORMATION

Warfarin – INR – 2.3 on x/xx/xx

PHARMACY ONLY	INITIAL AND DATE
Clinical Check in dispensary	SP x/xx
Clinical Check at ward level by CP	PNEG x/xx
Labelled/Dispensed	
Checked	
Medication Card Required	

Comments
All medications reconciled on discharge by a clinical pharmacist Y or N

Prescribed by J James PIP 3357
Pharmacist Independent Prescriber

(Signature)   ....
GMC Number

Date:
Grade:
Bleep No:

Figure 2.7—cont'd

Abbreviations for frequency

Once daily	= od	Every morning	= om or mane
Twice daily	= bd	Every night	= on or nocte
Three times daily	= tds or tid		
Four times daily	= qds or qid		

As Required Medicines
Check for allergies / drug sensitivities

Medicine Paracetamol			Start Date x/xx	Date	x/x														
Dose 1 g	Route O	Freq. (max) 4-6 hrly	Stop Date	Time	10:00														
Signature *S.Logger*			Signature	Dose Route	1g O														
Special Instructions / Directions * Max 8 daily *			Pharmacy PP	Given by	SL														
Medicine			Start Date	Date															
Dose	Route	Freq. (max)	Stop Date	Time															
Signature			Signature	Dose Route															
Special Instructions / Directions			Pharmacy	Given by															
Medicine			Start Date	Date															
Dose	Route	Freq. (max)	Stop Date	Time															
Signature			Signature	Dose Route															
Special Instructions / Directions			Pharmacy	Given by															
Medicine			Start Date	Date															
Dose	Route	Freq. (max)	Stop Date	Time															
Signature			Signature	Dose Route															
Special Instructions / Directions			Pharmacy	Given by															
Medicine			Start Date	Date															
Dose	Route	Freq. (max)	Stop Date	Time															
Signature			Signature	Dose Route															
Special Instructions / Directions			Pharmacy	Given by															
Medicine			Start Date	Date															
Dose	Route	Freq. (max)	Stop Date	Time															
Signature			Signature	Dose Route															
Special Instructions / Directions			Pharmacy	Given by															

Omitted Doses of Medication

Date	Time	Medication, Dose and Route	Reason for omission and action taken	Signature

Figure 2.8—cont'd

The Hospital

DR NAME + ADDRESS
                    GP CODE:

Patient Name	Jenny Richardson
Patient Address	11 Tae Avenue

Admission Date:	**30/06/2016**	Phone No:	**02890666666**
Admission Method:	**Via A&E**	DOB:	5/12/69 Age: 47
Discharge Date:		Sex:	**M /Ⓕ**(delete as applicable)
Discharge Method:	**Discharge to home**	H&C No:	Missing
Ward:	**Ward One**		
Discharging Consultant:	**Dr. Pantridge**		

CURRENT EPISODE DETAILS

Principal Diagnosis:	Twisted ankle
Underlying Conditions & Co-Morbidities:	Bipolar
Procedures/Dates:	
Relevant clinical concerns:	Pain control

FOLLOW UP PLANS	COMMENTS
Outstanding Investigations:	N/A
Hospital Review Arrangements:	N/A
Additional Care Arrangements:	N/A
Action Required By GP:	Review pain in 1 week

Figure 2.9   Jenny Richardson's discharge prescription (for OSCE 2.5)

Continued

ALLERGY/DRUG SENSITIVITIES	NKDA			TYPE OF REACTION (IF KNOWN)			

MEDICATION ON DISCHARGE

Take home supply needed Y/N	MEDICINE (APPROVED NAME)	ROUTE	DOSE AND FREQUENCY	NOTES / COMMENTS DURATION IF APPROPRIATE, INDICATION IF NEW DRUG, TITRATION ETC.	CHANGES N-New I-Increased D-Decreased	PHARMACY INFORMATION (INCLUDING QUANTITY SUPPLIED)
Y	Lithium	0	400 mg mane	Ongoing	—	—
Y	Simvastatin	0	40 mg nocte	Ongoing	—	—
Y	Paracetamol	0	1 g 4-6 hourly	x 5 days	—	—

MEDICATION STOPPED	REASON FOR STOPPING

ADDITIONAL MEDICATION INFORMATION

PHARMACY ONLY	INITIAL AND DATE
Clinical Check in dispensary	P.P. x/xx/xx
Clinical Check at ward level by CP	
Labelled/Dispensed	
Checked	
Medication Card Required	

Comments
All medications reconciled on discharge by a clinical pharmacist Y or N

Prescribed by J Smith PIP 3357
Pharmacist Independent Prescriber

Date:
Grade:
Bleep No:

(Signature)   ....
GMC Number

Figure 2.9—cont'd

OSCE Answer sheet (for OSCE 2.5)

Candidate name:		Date:	

State safety, legal or accuracy issue:	State how you would resolve this issue:

OSCE Mark sheet (for OSCE 2.1)

Candidate's Name		Date	

Assessment Criteria for example 2.1:	Mark		
Accuracy and legal check:			
1. Identifies that the simvastatin should be labelled 'one to be taken at night' instead of 'one to be taken as directed'.	0	1	–
Clinical check:			
2. *Identifies an interaction between statin and itraconazole – avoid use together as per BNF and Stockley.*	0	–	4
3. Identifies issue with interaction: itraconazole is a potent inhibitor of CYP3A4 and exposure will affect metabolism and lead to raised simvastatin levels (1 mark). Raised statin concentrations are known to be associated with the development of myopathy and rhabdomyolysis (1 mark).	0	1	2
4. Action – contact GP to highlight the problem.	0	1	
5. If a short course of an azole is considered essential, the statin manufacturers suggest temporary withdrawal of the statin (from Stockley).	0	1	
6. Tinea corporis can be treated over 15 or 7 days – student should suggest a 200 mg BD for 7 days and holding the statin.	0	1	
Any other valid point up to a maximum of 2 points e.g.			
7. Mentions counselling points for patient on statin e.g. muscle pain	0	1	2
8. Stopping statin for 7-day treatment			
9. Counselling the patient regarding possible hepatotoxicity			
10. Preventing spread of fungal infection e.g. avoid sharing towels			
11. Do not scratch e.g. reducing chance of secondary infection			
Issue(s) relating to patient safety:			
If candidates propose any course of action which could lead to serious harm or death, they will **fail** the OSCE. Always seek a second opinion. Give detail:			

Total Mark:	/12 (max)	
Angoff score: 6 Criterion in bold italics is essential (criterion 2)	**Pass**	**Fail**

Assessors Comments:

Assessor's Signature: _____

OSCE Mark sheet (for OSCE 2.2)

Candidate's Name		Date	

Assessment Criteria for example 2.2:	Mark		
Accuracy and legal check:			
1. Identifies that the prescription is not coded.	0	1	–
2. Identifies that the label for the Camcolit® does not contain all of the necessary warnings **(25 missing).**	0	1	
Clinical check			
3. *Identifies that there is an interaction between the lithium and the diclofenac.*	0	–	5
4. NSAIDs can increase lithium levels leading to toxicity.	0	1	
5. Stockley states: most NSAIDs should be avoided, especially if other risk factors are present.	0	1	
6. Avoid unless serum lithium levels can be very well monitored (initially every few days) and the dose reduced appropriately.	0	1	
7. Notify GP and discuss possibility of maintaining paracetamol alone for short term pain	0	1	
Any other valid point up to a maximum of 2 points e.g.			
8. Student may state that other medications taken by the patient should be checked for suitability with lithium.	0	1	2
9. Student may state that patient should have a lithium card.			
10. Student may state that patient should receive counselling regarding adequate fluid intake, avoid increase or decrease in sodium intake.			
11. Student may state that patient should be warned about buying OTC analgesics.			
12. Student may state that patient should be counselled on toxicity e.g. lethargy, drowsiness etc.			
13. Student may advise patient to see GP again for additional suitable analgesia if paracetamol is inadequate.			
Issue(s) relating to patient safety:			
If candidates propose any course of action which could lead to serious harm or death, they will **fail** the OSCE. Always seek a second opinion. Give detail: _____ _____			

Total Mark:	**/13 (max)**	
Angoff score: 7 Criterion in bold italics is essential (criterion 3)	**Pass**	**Fail**

Assessors Comments:

Assessor's Signature: _____

OSCE station mark sheet (for OSCE 2.3)

Candidate's Name		Date	

Issues correctly identified and suggested changes to practice	Mark			
Dispensing issues				
1. *The individual dose on Epanutin label is wrong (6 mL on label should be 8 mL).*	0	–	–	5
2. Product labelled for Doublebase emollient bath additive instead of Doublebase Dayleve gel.	0	–	2	–
Suggestions for changes to practice – may suggest any of the following or other reasonable alternative.				
3. Encourage dispensers to double check own work.	0	1		
4. Training for staff on calculations.				
5. Always get another member of pharmacy team to double check calculations.				
6. Review of understanding of relevant SOPs in the pharmacy.				
Issue(s) relating to patient safety:				
If candidates propose any course of action which could lead to serious harm or death, they will **fail** the OSCE. Always seek a second opinion. Give detail: _____ _____				

Total Mark:	/8 (max)	
Angoff score: 5 Criterion in bold italics is essential (criterion 1)	**Pass**	**Fail**

Assessors Comments:

Assessor's Signature: _____

OSCE Mark sheet (for OSCE 2.4)

Candidate's Name		Date		

Assessment Criteria for example 2.4:	Mark		
Legal Prescription Requirements			
1. Identifies that prescription is **not** signed.	0	–	2
2. Contacts prescriber to arrange getting the prescription signed.	0	–	2
Accuracy issues with prescription			
3. Indicates on answer sheet that date of birth is **missing** from the prescription.	0	–	2
4. Prescriber or pharmacist to add date of birth.	0	1	–
5. Indicates on answer sheet that medicines are prescribed generically.	0	1	–
Safety issues with prescription			
6. Identifies that there is a drug interaction between ibuprofen and warfarin **(1 mark)** where the anticoagulant effect is possibly enhanced **(1 mark)**.	0	1	2
7. Identifies that ibuprofen (or NSAIDs) are associated with serious GI toxicity **(1 mark)** and that there is a possible increased bleeding risk with warfarin **(1 mark)**.	0	1	2
8. *Prescriber to stop ibuprofen.*	0	–	2
9. Prescriber to add paracetamol / codeine to prescription.	0	1	–
DiscretionaryAny other valid point (i.e. only awarded if full marks not obtained elsewhere)			
10. NSAID use can be associated with a small increased risk of thrombotic events.	0	1	2
11. INR monitoring / range			
Suggests completing incident form.			
Other_____			
Issue(s) relating to patient safety			
If candidates propose any course of action which could lead to serious harm or death, they will **fail** the OSCE. Always seek a second opinion. Give detail: _____ _____			

Total Mark:	/15 (max)	
Angoff Score: 7 Criterion in bold italics is essential (criterion 8)	Pass	Fail

Assessors Comments:

Assessor's Signature: _____

OSCE Mark sheet (for OSCE 2.5)

Candidate's Name		Date	

Assessment Criteria for example 2.5:	Mark		
Legal Prescription Requirements			
1. Identifies that prescription is **not** signed.	0	–	2
2. Contacts prescriber to arrange getting prescription signed.	0	–	2
Accuracy issues with prescription			
3. Indicates on answer sheet that H&C (or hospital) number is **missing** from the prescription.	0	–	2
4. Prescriber or pharmacist to add H&C (or hospital) number.	0	1	–
Safety and efficacy issues with prescription			
5. Identifies lithium has been prescribed generically **(1 mark)** and brand prescribing is indicated as preparations vary widely in bioavailability (BNF) **(1 mark).**	0	1	2
6. *Prescriber to change to Camcolit 400 mg tablets in the morning / once daily*	0	–	2
DiscretionaryAny other valid point (i.e. only awarded if full marks not obtained elsewhere)			
Requests / checks lithium level	0	1	2
Lithium range: 0.4–1 mmol/L			
Suggests review of analgesia requirements			
Suggests completing incident form			
Other_____			
Issue(s) relating to patient safety			
If candidates propose any course of action which could lead to serious harm or death, they will **fail** the OSCE. Always seek a second opinion. Give detail: _____			

Total Mark:	/11 (max)	
Angoff Score: 6 Criterion in bold italics is essential (criterion 6)	Pass	Fail

Assessors Comments:

Assessor's Signature: _____

✓ How to excel in this type of station

Action	Reason	How
Be systematic	To ensure you don't miss anything and to maintain patient safety, follow your checking procedure.	Systematically review the prescription for legal, clinical and transcription errors.
Suggest resolutions to any errors identified	Whilst it is essential to identify any errors, you need to provide suggestions/resolutions to the problems encountered.	Consider what the best outcome for the patient would be e.g. if you identify that the dose is too low for the patient's indication, body surface area and renal function, suggest the appropriate dose and where you found this information.

✗ Common errors in this type of station

Action	Remedy	Reason
Not identifying clinical issues	Read the task and the prescription carefully. Pay particular attention to the medical history and medication history and check that all required medicines are prescribed, as per evidence based medicine and at the correct dose / frequency for their intended indication.	To ensure that the prescription is accurate from a clinical perspective and to reduce the risk to the patient from sub-therapeutic dosing or inappropriate drug choice.
Not identifying legal errors	For example; a prescription could be unsigned making it invalid – check both the medication kardex and the prescription for a prescriber's signature.	The prescriber may have been interrupted prior to completing the task – there may be omitted medication; the medication may not have been written by a prescriber. Medication cannot be administered to a patient without a valid prescriber's signature.

Further reading

Medicines Governance Northern Ireland: Medicine Safety Matters, Vol 3, Issue 1. <http://www.medicinesgovernance.hscni.net/wpfb-file/150211medicines-safetymatterscpvol3issue1-pdf> (accessed 14.10.15).

Royal Pharmaceutical Society: Medicines, Ethics and Practice Guide 39. <http://www.rpharms.com/support/mep.asp> (accessed 14.10.15).

National Pharmacy Association. <https://www.npa.co.uk/Knowledge-Centre/Publications/?cat=503&page=2> (accessed 14.10.15).

Background

Community pharmacists are required to deal with patients and their symptoms on a daily basis. Pharmacists may recommend a product or treatment with an appropriate evidence base, give advice or indeed refer the patient to an alternative healthcare professional.

The consultation with the patient requires pharmacists to use all of their communication skills to help make a differential diagnosis.

Differential diagnosis: the determination of which of two or more diseases with similar symptoms is the one from which the patient is suffering, by a systematic comparison and contrasting of the clinical findings. – Farlex Partner Medical Dictionary 2012

Different pharmacy courses will teach and assess this skill at different levels. At some point in your course you will have been taught and practised the necessary communication skills of the consultation and mnemonics may have been used initially to help you with the process. A mnemonic can help pharmacists to gather the information to help them make differential diagnoses. However, you must be cautious when using a mnemonic because a mnemonic may not contain all necessary information that is needed to make an accurate final diagnosis and further questioning may be needed depending on how a patient responds to your questions. Remember to listen to the answers from your patient and consider these carefully!

'Listen to the patient, he is telling you the diagnosis'—Sir William Osler, 1904

Popular mnemonics include:

ASMETHOD	
A	Age/appearance
S	Self or someone else
M	Medication
E	Extra medicines
T	Time persisting
H	History
O	Other symptoms
D	Danger symptoms
SIT DOWN, SIR	
S	Site or location of a sign/symptom
I	Intensity or severity

Continued

T	Type or nature
D	Duration
O	Onset
W	With (other symptoms)
N	Annoyed or aggravated by
S	Spread or radiation
I	Incidence or frequency
R	Relieved by

You can improve your overall communication skills through observing others and most importantly practising these skills through class exercises, with fellow students or with patients on placement. Make the most of these opportunities to ask for feedback from your peers and indeed patients. How did you come across to the patient?

Communication skills include:

• Verbal and non-verbal communication
• Tone of voice
• Your facial expressions
• Body language

In an OSCE scenario the consultation may well take place at a desk, so therefore you may have limited control over your environment, but you can still control how you communicate and come across to the patient. Marks will normally be awarded for your communication skills and it is important to practise and become comfortable with speaking with the patient. There are a number of excellent resources for responding to symptoms which have been listed in the reference section. Your own course may have used a core text or resource which can be used in the following OSCE stations.

Preparation

You are not expected to learn and regurgitate large volumes of information for this type of assessment. Most competency-based assessments will provide relevant reference texts or resources where information can be found.

How to have a consultation with a patient

There will be at least one station that involves an interaction with a patient. As part of your MPharm course you may have counselled using the Calgary-Cambridge model (see Figure 3.1). You can employ this again when counselling your patient at the verbal station. In the verbal station you should take time to prepare what you want to say and make notes on this beforehand.

How to use station resources

All of the resources you will need will be present at the station. Remember, if there is a resource at the station it most likely is needed to complete the task correctly! All products will come with patient information sheets or SPCs. Remember, in a patient consultation the patient is the most important resource. Pay attention to how they act and the responses that they give.

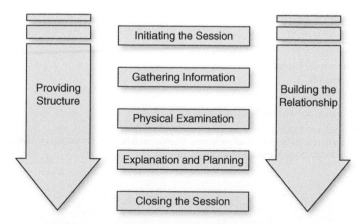

Figure 3.1 The Calgary-Cambridge model. Source: Kurtz SM et al 2003.

Buddy activity

When you see the Buddy sign you will need to pair up with a partner so that your partner can act out the role of the patient

---

Example 3.1.   OSCE Examination

Community Pharmacy Interaction

Please read the following information carefully. You have 10 minutes to complete the task.

Background

It is Monday morning and you are the responsible pharmacist on duty in a community pharmacy. You are asked to speak with a woman who is planning a holiday to the Island of Luzon in the Philippines. She is not known to you. The patient has been referred to you by the local practice nurse for malaria prophylaxis advice. The local practice nurse has already dealt with the vaccination requirements and given the patient advice on bite-avoidance measures.

Task

1. Introduce yourself and speak with the patient

2. Advise the patient appropriately on the antimalarial regimen required for her destination

You are provided with resources for the consultation, including the patient. The station supervisor will play the part of the patient – let the supervisor know when you are ready to speak with the patient.

Please submit your answer sheet to the examiner at the end of the OSCE and do not forget to include your name on the form.

DO NOT write on or remove any materials provided.

Station props that would be provided

Item required

1. Instructions for candidate.

2. Candidate answer sheet.

3. Candidate mark sheet.

4. NPA leaflet on malaria prophylaxis or access to NaTHNaC website.

5. chloroquine, proguanil, combi pack.

6. NaTHNaC leaflet on bite avoidance for patient.

NaTHNaC = National Travel Health Network & Centre.
NB: the requirements for anti-malarial regimens change on a regular basis please consult the most up-to-date guidance before making a recommendation.

OSCE Station – Script for patient actor (for OSCE 3.1)

Your name is Mandy Stevens. You are 41 years old and heading out to the Island of Luzon in the Philippines in June this year with your husband to celebrate your 20th wedding anniversary.

You will be staying in the Luzon Marriott Resort & Spa for 3 weeks.

OSCE station – Patient actor's brief

You want to know if you need antimalarial tablets for your holiday with your husband.

If asked where you are travelling to say ...

'Island of Luzon in the Philippines.'

If asked for how long say ...

'We are heading away for 3 weeks at the start of June.'

If asked about where you are staying say ...

'We are staying in a 5 star hotel, the Luzan Marriott, we got a great deal.'

If asked if you are planning any day trips or cruises say ...

'No.'

If asked if you are planning to stay within the same country say ...

'Yes.'

If asked who exactly is travelling say ...

'Myself and my husband.'

If asked about your age say ...

'41.'

If asked about your husband's age say ...

'He is 47 years old.'

OSCE Station – Script for patient actor (for OSCE 3.1)—cont'd

If asked about medical condition/health say …

'I am very healthy, I don't suffer from anything.'

If asked about your husband's medical conditions/health say …

'He has a heart condition, something to do with an irregular heartbeat.'

If you are asked about your medication say …

'I don't take any medication, just the odd paracetamol for a headache.'

If you are asked about your husband's medication say …

'My husband takes amiodarone tablets daily for his heart condition.'

If you are asked about vaccinations say …

'We have both attended the practice nurse last week to get vaccinations and she gave us some information on insect bites'. YOU CAN SHOW THE CANDIDATE THE INFORMATION LEAFLET GIVEN TO YOU BY THE NURSE.

If you are asked about pregnancy or breast feeding say …

'No, I am not pregnant or breast feeding.'

If asked if you have any questions say …

'No, I will come back tomorrow and get everything that I need.'

OSCE Answer sheet (for OSCE 3.1)

Candidate name:		Date:	

Use the space below to make any notes before you counsel the patient.

✔ How to excel in this type of station

Action	Reason	How
Be systematic	You will need vital information before making a recommendation, including a full medication history and exact details about accommodation etc.	NPA documents list questions for patients in this position and highlight the medicines which could interact with anti-malarials. Remember to use your resources!

✘ Common errors in this type of station

Action	Remedy	Reason
Not identifying clinical issues	Read the task carefully and remember that most people do not travel alone. You need a medication history for <u>all</u> travellers in this scenario.	Patients sometimes assume that medication bought over the counter carry fewer risks than prescription only medicines however you need a full medication history before selling this type of medication.

👥 Buddy activity

Example 3.2. OSCE Examination

OSCE Station: Making a differential diagnosis

Background

It is Monday morning and you are the pharmacist on duty in a community pharmacy. You are asked by your assistant to talk to a customer (Melanie Keenan) who wants some advice on her daughter's (Jenny) symptoms. She is not known to you.

Task

1. Take a history.

2. Attempt to make an assessment of the probable cause of her problem (definitive diagnosis).

3. In the examination situation you might be asked by the examiner what your assessment of the patient's problem is.

You are provided with resources for the consultation, including the patient. The station supervisor will play the part of the patient – let the supervisor know when you are ready to speak with the patient.

Please submit your answer sheet to the examiner at the end of the OSCE and do not forget to include your name on the form.

DO NOT write on or remove any materials provided.

Station props that would be provided

Item required

1. Instructions for candidate.

2. Candidate answer sheet.

3. Candidate mark sheet.

4. Patient script.

5. Copy of Rutter – Community pharmacy or alternative pharmacy text book/resource.

6. Photograph of rash (Figure 3.2).

Figure 3.2 Skin rash (for OSCE 3.2).

OSCE Station – Script for patient actor (for OSCE 3.2)

It is Monday morning and you are in the local community pharmacy asking for help about your daughter's symptoms. Your daughter's name is Jenny. The assistant at the counter has referred you to the pharmacist, who you do not know. You can respond to the pharmacist's questions using the information below.

You are Melanie Keenan, aged 22

Your daughter Jenny is 3 years old and has just started nursery school.

Her symptoms began last night when she:

* Complained of feeling tired

* Refused to eat her dinner.

She has since developed a temperature of 38° C.

If asked about a rash or any other symptoms you can show the student the image below.

There are a few very small spots which have appeared on her back this morning and they seem to be itchy.

She is not currently taking or using any medication.

You have not tried anything yet.

Additional information:

The skin surrounding the blisters is not red and/or painful.

There is no pain in the chest or difficulty breathing.

There are no signs of dehydration, such as drowsiness and cold hands and feet.

There are no major warning symptoms indicating complications e.g. confusion, stiff neck, vomiting, behavioural changes, ataxia, seizures etc.

Melanie is not overly concerned about Jenny but would like to rule out anything serious.

Patient photograph shows small, red spots, most of which have developed a blister on top.

OSCE Answer sheet (for OSCE 3.2)

Candidate name:		Date:	

Use the space below to make any notes before you interview the patient.

Differential diagnosis:

OSCE station mark sheet (for OSCE 3.1)

Candidate's Name		Date	

Assessment criteria:	Mark			
1. Introduces himself or herself, including name **(1 mark)** and position **(1 mark)**	0	1	2	-
2. Checks exact location for travel	0	1		
3. Checks who exactly is travelling	0	1		
4. Checks length of stay	0	1		
5. Checks ages of both travellers **(2 marks if both checked)**	0	1	2	-
6. Checks current medications for both travellers **(2 marks if both checked)**	0	1	2	-
7. Checks medical conditions for both travellers **(2 marks if both checked)**	0	1	2	-
8. Checks for pregnancy and breast feeding	0	1		
9. Checks if taking day trips or cruises or travelling elsewhere	0	1		
10. Final recommendation				4
• Refers Mandy's husband to the GP as the chloroquine is contraindicated with his amiodarone				
• Mandy requires proguanil two tablets daily plus chloroquine 2 tabs weekly. Needs 8 weeks of treatment. (i.e., 1 week before, whilst there and for 4 weeks after returning)				2
11. Patient can be reminded about ensuring bite avoidance measures as discussed with the practice nurse	0			1
12. See doctor immediately if ill within 1 year **(1 mark)**, esp. 3 months after return **(1 mark)**	0	1	2	
13. Asks patient if she has any questions	0	1	-	-
If candidates propose any course of action which could compromise patient safety, they will **fail** the OSCE.	**Pass**		**Fail**	

Professionalism including communication style

Excellent	**All of the time:** appropriately attentive with patient: empathetic and interested: identifies and resolves problems e.g. if patient drinks or smokes attempted health promotion: doesn't cause embarrassment or loss of face to patient: checks patient understanding by asking patient to repeat back (counselling) or repeating back (history taking), organised questioning/provision of information: body language appropriate & eye contact good.	4
Good	**Most of the time** (as above).	3
Average	**Some of the time** (as above).	2
Poor	**Most of the time:** inattentive with patient: lack of empathy and interest: lack of problem identification or resolution: causes embarrassment or loss of face to patient: omitted check of patient understanding by asking patient to repeat back (counselling) or repeating back (history taking), disorganised questioning/provision of information: body language inappropriate & eye contact poor.	1
Fail	**All of the time** (as above).	0

Continued

OSCE station mark sheet (for OSCE 3.1)—cont'd

Total Mark:		/27	
Angoff: 16 – criterion in bold italics is essential to pass this OSCE Recommendation (tick most appropriate term):		Fail	Pass

Assessor's comments

Assessor's signature_____

OSCE station mark sheet (for OSCE 3.2)

Candidate's Name		Date		

Assessment criteria:	Mark			
1. Introduce themselves including name **(1 mark)** and position **(1 mark)**	0	1	2	-
2. Explains the purpose of the discussion	0	1	-	-
3. Asks Melanie if the advice is for her daughter	0	1	-	-
4. Checks the age of the patient	0	1		-
5. Checks medication (1) – if she has tried anything already (1)	0	1	2	-
6. Checks time persisting	0	1	-	-
7. Checks history and assesses				
• Raised temperature	0	1		
• Loss of appetite	0	1		
• Itchy red spots	0	1		
• Blister on top	0	1		
• Located in her back	0	1		
• No secondary infection	0	1		
• No signs of dehydration	0	1		
• No respiratory distress or other warning symptoms	0	1		
8. Checks if there are other warning symptoms	0	1		-
9. Thanks the patient for her time/help	0	1	-	-
10. Makes the correct differential diagnosis as chickenpox	0	5	-	-
If candidates propose any course of action which could compromise patient safety, they will **fail** the OSCE.	**Pass**		**Fail**	

OSCE station mark sheet (for OSCE 3.2)—cont'd

Professionalism including communication style

Excellent	**All of the time:** appropriately attentive with patient: empathetic and interested: identifies and resolves problems e.g. if patient drinks or smokes attempted health promotion: doesn't cause embarrassment or loss of face to patient: checks patient understanding by asking patient to repeat back (counselling) or repeating back (history taking), organised questioning/ provision of information: body language appropriate & eye contact good.	4
Good	**Most of the time (as above).**	3
Average	**Some of the time (as above).**	2
Poor	**Most of the time:** inattentive with patient: lack of empathy and interest: lack of problem identification or resolution: causes embarrassment or loss of face to patient: omitted check of patient understanding by asking patient to repeat back (counselling) or repeating back (history taking), disorganised questioning/provision of information: body language inappropriate & eye contact poor.	1
Fail	**All of the time (as above).**	0

Total Mark:		/27	
Angoff score (borderline competence): 11 Criterion in bold italics is essential to pass this OSCE (criterion 10). Recommendation (tick most appropriate term):		**Fail**	**Pass**

Assessor's comments:

Assessor's signature_____

Further reading

Kurtz, S., Silverman, J., Benson, J., Draper, J., 2003. Marrying content and process in clinical method teaching: enhancing the calgary-cambridge guides. Acad. Med. 78 (8), 802–809.

National Travel Health Network & Centre (NaTHNaC). Retrieved 8 September 2015 from <http://travelhealthpro.org.uk>.

NHS Choices. Retrieved 8 September 2015 from <http://www.nhs.uk/Conditions/Chickenpox/Pages/Complications.aspx>.

Rutter, P., 2013. Community pharmacy, symptoms, diagnosis and treatment, 3rd ed. Churchill Livingstone Elsevier.

4

The aim of this chapter is to provide you with the basic knowledge and understanding to successfully incorporate medication reconciliation, which includes medication history taking, in your daily practice and to participate effectively in a medication history OSCE.

Every time patients are transferred from one healthcare setting to another (for example, from home to hospital and vice versa) it is essential that accurate and reliable information about each patient's medication is transferred at the same time. This enables the multi-professional team responsible for the patient during admission or on discharge home to establish a complete picture of previously taken medications. It also supports future decisions regarding therapy for the next stage in the patient's medicines-management journey. For the purposes of this chapter, we will focus on the patient's admission to hospital.

This process is called *medicines reconciliation* and it is one of the basic principles of good medicines management. It should occur within 24 hours of the patient's admission to hospital.

Medicines reconciliation can be described in two discrete stages:

Stage 1: basic reconciliation (medication history)

This involves the collection of an accurate current list of the patient's medications. Ideally this should include details of all medicines the patient has tried in the past, however for most hospital admissions, it is usually sufficient to document the details of current prescribed and purchased medications as well as recently discontinued medications (for example courses of antibiotics, corticosteroids) along with details of any medication allergies and adverse reactions.

Stage 2: full reconciliation

This builds on Stage 1 and involves the healthcare professional taking the established list of current prescribed as well as purchased medications and comparing it to existing prescriptions for the patient, identifying any discrepancies between the two lists and then acting on that information to resolve the potential errors appropriately. In this process, it is important to consider the patient's reason for admission and current medical state when making decisions regarding the continuation of medications or their permanent or temporary withdrawal. All suggestions and decisions regarding medications should be documented appropriately in the patient's multi-professional notes so that all team members are aware. See Figure 4.1 which highlights the movement of information in relation to medication use for an individual patient.[1]

Goal of medicines reconciliation

The ultimate goal of medicines reconciliation is to prevent adverse drug events at all interfaces of patient care. Interfaces of patient care include:

- Admission to hospital/nursing home/care facility
- Transfer – from one ward to another, from one facility to another
- Discharge – to home/nursing home/care facility.

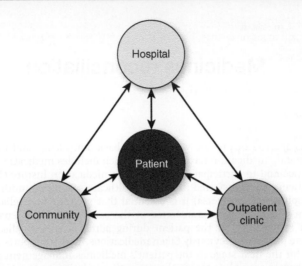

Figure 4.1 Patient and multi-professional interfaces in the medication information transfer process.

Medicines reconciliation aims to eliminate all undocumented intentional discrepancies as well as unintentional discrepancies by reconciling all medicines at all interfaces of care (see Fig. 4.2).

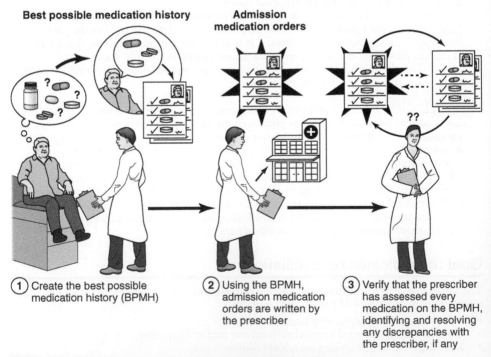

① Create the best possible medication history (BPMH)

② Using the BPMH, admission medication orders are written by the prescriber

③ Verify that the prescriber has assessed every medication on the BPMH, identifying and resolving any discrepancies with the prescriber, if any

Figure 4.2 PROACTIVE medication reconciliation model at admission.

An *undocumented intentional discrepancy* can occur when a prescriber deliberately or intentionally adds, changes or discontinues a medicine which the patient was taking prior to admission but does not clearly document this in the patient's medical record.

For example:

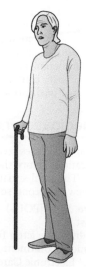

Mrs Parsa is admitted via Accident and Emergency following a fainting episode. She has all of her medicines with her in her handbag including her recently increased blood pressure medication, ramipril, now at a dose of 7.5 mg daily (previously 5 mg daily). (see Figure 4.3)

The admitting junior doctor decides to deliberately lower the dose of ramipril back to 5 mg daily, but doesn't note this in her medical notes. On admission to the Medical Ward later in the day, the patient is prescribed ramipril 7.5 mg daily.

Figure 4.3 Mrs Parsa.

An *unintentional discrepancy* can occur when the prescriber unintentionally changes, adds or omits a medicine which the patient was taking prior to admission.

For example:

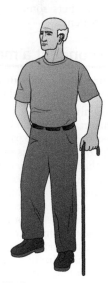

Mr Jameson is admitted to the surgical ward for a planned surgical procedure. He has taken some, but not all of his medication with him – he left his inhalers and his insulin at home as he doesn't really think about them as medication. (see Figure 4.4)

The admitting junior doctor writes up all of the medication which Mr Jameson brought with him, but does not include the inhalers or insulin as they are not present.

Figure 4.4 Mr Jameson.

Prevention of medication errors

Types of medication errors that can be prevented by reconciling medications may include:

- Failure to prescribe clinically important home medications while in hospital
- Incorrect doses or dosage forms
- Missed or duplicated doses resulting from inaccurate medication records
- Failure to clearly indicate which pre-admission medications should be resumed and/or discontinued after discharge from hospital
- Duplication of therapy at the point of discharge – for example due to brand and generic forms co-prescribed, combination preparations, pre-admission medications prescribed alongside altered medications

Taking a medication history

When conducting medicines reconciliation, the first step is to obtain an accurate medication history. A medication history should ideally be taken within 24 hours of the patient's admission to hospital. The ideal situation for the most accurate medication history should include a patient interview. A second source is always required. This could include:

1. Patient's own drugs (PODs)
2. GP repeat list
3. A copy of a discharge letter from another hospital (recent – within one month)
4. A recent clinic appointment medication list
5. Access to the Electronic Care Record and GP information
6. A family member or carer's information
7. Community pharmacy records
8. GP letter
9. Dosette box.

The guide below offers some suggestions to support you when conducting a medication history with a patient.

How to ... conduct a medication history (the patient interview)

Note: This guide deals only with interviewing the patient to obtain a medication history. In practice at least two sources would be required e.g. GP surgery record, patient's own medicines.

1. Before you start:
    a. It is important to obtain background information in relation to the patient's reason for admission. Review the past medical history, social history and any medication histories already completed. This may help you jog patients' memories when speaking to them.
    b. Assess that patients are appropriate to interview or if they have any communication challenges including speech or hearing deficiencies or if they require an interpreter.
2. Talk to the patient, for example, ask the patient:
    a. To tell you about all the medications they currently take, including vaccinations
    b. If they are responsible for taking and storing their own medications or if they have a carer
    c. Where they obtain their medicines e.g. if they have a regular pharmacy who may help to fill in gaps if necessary
3. Patient list as a medication history source
    The patient may hand you a list of medicines or attempt to tell you all the medicines they take. The accuracy of this will vary from patient to patient and the number of

medicines they take. Unfortunately the majority of patients won't give you **all** the possible information. You may then have to prompt them further to find out the complete list of medicines.

4. What detail do you require regarding the medication?
   a. All prescribed medications
   b. Name, strength, dosing schedule and duration.
   c. Prompt the patient further about specific forms other than oral e.g. inhaled, patches, injections, eye/ear drops, topical etc. Sometimes patients don't view these types of drugs as medicines.
   d. Probe further if required regarding how often they take 'as required' medication and if they are taking all their medicines as prescribed (adherence).
   e. Always ask patients if they require any medicines supplied directly from a hospital e.g. specialist medicines are often not supplied via GP/community pharmacist.
5. Over the counter (OTC) and complementary medications
   Ask about OTC and complementary therapies e.g. herbal, homeopathic, which they may have obtained in the pharmacy/in a supermarket/online. These medicines may have caused admission or may interact with other prescribed medication.
6. Determine allergy and/or sensitivity status
   If patient confirms they have allergies, always check what the reaction was e.g. rash, swollen tongue. Some patients confuse allergy with intolerance e.g. nausea due to an antibiotic.
7. Ask about previous adverse drug reactions (ADRs) to medications e.g. angiotensin-converting enzyme inhibitor–induced cough or statin-induced muscle pain.
8. Ask about any recent changes to their medication (either commenced or ceased) as this may enable you to pick up drug-related admissions.

To further support your development of this clinical skill, we have put together a sample interview (see below under 'sample patient interview') which provides suggestions for how you might structure an interview with a patient and how you might phrase the questions you need to ask in order to gain the best information from your patient. An example of the type of form you might use to record this information can be found in Figure 4.5.

Buddy activity

Sample patient interview

The following are suggested questions when carrying out a patient interview. You may not need to ask all of these questions or you may want to rephrase them.

It is good practice to use 'open' questions that allow the patients to demonstrate their understanding about their medicines, rather than 'direct' or 'leading' questions.

Introduction

'Hello. My name is _____ and I'm a 1st/2nd/3rd/4th–year pharmacy student on the ward/clinic. Could you tell me your name?'

'Thank you, _____. I'd like to ask you some questions about the medicines that you regularly take at home, is it a good time to talk to you?'

'That's great, thank you. I need to ask you some questions about the medicines that you took at home before you came in, would that be okay? It's important that we have a complete list of your medicines so that we can make the right decisions about your therapy while you are with us'

'Do you look after your own medication at home?'

Medicines Reconciliation Form	Name of student:

Date Patient initials TK DOB 5-9-1972 Hospital number CAH12345 Gender M	Date admitted	Tick sources used for medication history

Allergies/Drug sensitivities

Allergen/drug (generic name)	Type of reaction (e.g. rash)
....	....
....	....
....	....
....	....
Signature:	Date: ....

No known allergies

Signature: .... Date: ....

Past medical history: COPD Depression	Patient Patient Relative/carer GP surgery GP letter GP repeat list Emergency Care Summary Electronic care record Community Pharmacy Patients Own Drugs Patient medication list Medical notes Nursing/residential home list Recent discharge prescription Other: .....

Presenting complaint(s): SOB

Diagnosis: Exacerbation of COPD

Medication history confirmed (sign and date): F Davies

Medicines *prior* to admission

Medicine name, strength and form, route	Dose and frequency	Continued unchanged on admission	Altered on admission	Hold on admission	Stop on admission	Medicine omitted	Comments, notes
Budesonide (Pulmicort) Turbohaler 200 microgram (inhale)	2 puffs twice daily					✓	-
Terbutaline (Bricanyl) Turbohaler 500 microgram (inhale)	2 puffs twice daily when required					✓	-
Venlafaxine MR 150 mg capsule (oral)	One capsule at night	✓					-

Medicine(s) *added since* admission

Medicine name, strength and form, route *and date started*	Dose and frequency	Continues unchanged	Altered (date)	Held (date)	Stopped (date)	Comments, notes
Salbutamol CFC-free inhaler 100 microgram/inhalation	2 puffs when required, via Aerochamber	✓				-
Clarithromycin 500 mg tablet (oral)	-					No frequency nor duration on kardex
Salbutamol 2.5 mg nebules	2.5 mg when required	✓				-
Sodium chloride 0.9% nebules	2.5 ml when required	✓				-

From first being prescribed after admission to point where you check patient's kardex:

	GP details	Community pharmacy details	Height (m) ...1.65..... Weight (kg)....65..
			BMI (weight[kg]/height [m²]): **23.8**
name	Dr H. Fairley	Lipton's Pharmacy	
address	Fairley and Grainger Medical Practice, 70 Grosvenor Rd, Omagh	59 Grosvenor Rd, Omagh	Underweight <18.5 Ideal 18.5–25 Overweight 25–30
tel. number	02882 245678	02882 248765	Obese >30

Figure 4.5 An example of a Medicines Reconciliation form completed for a patient admitted with an exacerbation of COPD.

'Do you use a compliance aid such as a Dosette box or a Medi-Dose system?'
(If so) 'Do you fill it yourself or does someone help you with it?'
'Do you go to the same pharmacy all the time?........**(If so)** Which one?.....Would you mind if I contacted them if I need to clarify any information relating to your medicines?'
For patients who do not look after their own medications but a family member does (elderly, confused or paediatric patients):
'Would it be possible to discuss your regular medicines with a family member? How can we contact them?'
Medication allergies
'Are you allergic to any medications?'
(If so) 'What happened, what type of reaction did you have?'
Information gathering
'Are you taking any tablets that are prescribed for you by your family doctor or another doctor?'
(If so) 'Have you brought them with you?'*
If the patients have brought their medications with them, this is a good opportunity to check how the medicines are actually taken, by holding up each product and opening the packages. You also have the opportunity to check the date of dispensing and check about adherence.
(If the patient is prescribed medications but hasn't brought them in) 'Can you tell me their names, strengths and how many you take a day?'
You need to record information on each medication: the name, strength, dose, route, frequency, brand if appropriate. If the patient is taking the medication in a different way than the prescription indicates, it is important to record what the patient is actually taking, and note the discrepancy.
'Do you take any liquid medicines?'
'Do you use any inhalers to help your breathing?'
'Do you use any sprays or tablets which go under your tongue for chest pain?'
'Do you use any patches, drops, creams or ointments?'
'Does anyone give you any injections regularly including vaccines e.g. the flu vaccine? If so, what are they?'
OTC medicines/medicines from other sources
'Do you buy any medicines including herbal either from your pharmacy, supermarket, on-line or health food shop?'
'Do you buy any vitamins or minerals that you take regularly?'
'Do you use any other homeopathic or Chinese medicines?'
'Do you take any medicines that are supplied to you from a hospital?'
Record the details of all of these medications, dose, frequency, brand etc.
Medication-taking behaviour
'Have you commenced (any of the above types of medications) within the last month or two?'
'Have you stopped any medicines within the last 6 months? If so, why?'
'Do you take all your medicines as your doctor suggests or have you changed the doses of anything?'
'Have you ever had an unpleasant effect to any medicine? If so, what happened?'
You should close the patient interview by asking patients if they have any questions about their medicines, either those they have taken before they came into hospital or those they have been prescribed in hospital.
Thank the patient for their time.

*If the patient has brought their own medications or PODs with them into hospital, this can act as a second source for you to use when compiling your list for your medication history and for future reconciliation.

Summary

Medicines reconciliation is a process which has been designed to prevent medication errors at all interfaces of care (admission, transfer and discharge). It involves three steps:

1. Obtain the most complete and accurate list possible of the patient's regular medications (prescribed and purchased).
   a. A patient interview should always be included where possible.
   b. Always use more than one source to complete your history.
2. Use this list when writing a prescription for the patient.
3. Compare this list with all prescriptions including inpatient medication kardexes and discharge prescriptions in order to identify any discrepancies and to discuss these with the multi-professional team, documenting your findings in the patient notes.

Sample OSCEs

The clinical skill of taking and documenting an accurate medication history is essential for every pharmacist. This skill demonstrates your competence with communication skills (verbal and written), history taking, interpretation of information as well as counselling of patients on their medication (if appropriate), assessment of adherence and also having liaisons with other healthcare professionals to resolve medication-related problems, if appropriate.

We have included a number of medication history OSCE examples in this chapter for you to work through with your colleagues. All of the examples have associated scripts for the patient actors as well as marking schemes to assess your performance. Many schools of pharmacy will use a similar style of marking grid, including details of knowledge you must gain, as well as aspects of good communication and professionalism which you must display. We have included a table of details of how professionalism and communication may be judged to provide you with a guide.

Communication skills

During the verbal OSCE stations, you are assessed not only on your knowledge but also on your professionalism and communication style. Table 4.1 below gives you an idea of how this will be assessed by the examiner.

Table 4.1

Professionalism including communication style		
Excellent	**All of the time:** appropriately attentive with patient: empathetic and interested: identifies and resolves problems e.g. if patient drinks or smokes attempted health promotion: doesn't cause embarrassment or loss of face to patient: checks patient understanding by asking repeating back (history taking), organised questioning/provision of information: body language appropriate & eye contact good.	4
Good	**Most of the time (as above)**	3
Average	**Some of the time (as above)**	2
Poor	**Most of the time:** inattentive with patient: lack of empathy and interest: lack of problem identification or resolution: causes embarrassment or loss of face to patient: omitted check of patient understanding by repeating back (history taking), disorganised questioning/provision of information: body language inappropriate & eye contact poor.	1
Fail	**All of the time (as above)**	0

Mapping against General Pharmaceutical
Counsel (GPhC) competencies for education

We have mapped our medication histories against the GPhC competencies for initial education and training. See the table below for what is expected depending on the level a student is at in the MPharm course, as can be evaluated via a simulation in OSCE. We expect that medication history skill starts to be developed during the second year of a four-year course and then is continually built upon during the subsequent years. Knowledge of medication in the first year is usually not sufficient to support this skill, although degree courses may differ in this respect. See Table 4.2 for suggested competencies throughout the 4 year MPharm.

Table 4.2 GPhC competencies measured by this type of OSCE

		Second year	Third year	Fourth year
10.2.2 (g)	Communicate with patients about their prescribed treatment	Shows how	shows how	shows how
10.2.2 (i)	Record, maintain and store patient data	Knows how	shows how	shows how
10.2.4 (f)	Conclude consultation to ensure a satisfactory outcome	Knows how	shows how	shows how
10.2.4 (g)	Maintain accurate and comprehensive consultation records	Knows how	shows how	shows how
10.2.4 (h)	Provide accurate written or oral information appropriate to the needs of patients, the public or other healthcare professionals	Knows how	shows how	shows how
10.2.5 (a)	Demonstrate the characteristics of a prospective professional pharmacist as set out in relevant codes of conduct and behaviour	Shows how	Does	Does

👤 Buddy activity

Example 4.1. Fourth-Year OSCE Examination

OSCE Station – Medication History Taking

Please read the following information carefully. You have 10 minutes to complete the activity.

Background

It is a Saturday morning, and you are a pharmacist providing a weekend ward service.

You are working on the Medical Admissions Unit (MAU).

Mrs Siobhan O'Toole, a 39-year-old woman, has been admitted via A&E with a suspected right deep vein thrombosis (DVT) which is a 'blood clot' in the leg.

Past medical/surgical history:

- Hypothyroidism (underfunctioning thyroid gland)
- Iron deficiency anaemia (insufficient oxygen carrying capacity of blood)
- Appendicectomy (removal of appendix)

Activity

1. Establish Mrs O'Toole's medication history.

You are **NOT** required to decide if medicines should be stopped, withheld or started.

2. Document the medication history on the front page of the partially completed pharmaceutical care plan provided.

3. You are assessed on what you say to the patient as well as what you document on the pharmaceutical care plan.

You are provided with sources for the medication history, including the patient. There are two people seated at the station: the examiner and the patient. Introduce yourself to the patient when you are ready to begin.

Please submit your completed medication history to the examiner at the end of the OSCE and do not forget to include your name on the form.

DO NOT write on or remove the medication kardex or any other materials provided.

Station props that would be provided

Items required

1. Instructions for candidate.
2. Candidate answer sheet.
3. Page 1 of pharmaceutical care plan partially completed (Fig. 4.6).
4. Mark sheet.
5. BNF.
6. Labels for Siobhan O'Toole.
7. Script for patient actor.

Labels for prescription (for OSCE 4.1)

Keep out of reach and sight of children

28 Levothyroxine 100 mg tablets
Take ONE tablet DAILY
John O'Toole

Today's date · Name of pharmacy and address

Keep out of reach and sight of children

28 Ferrous fumarate 305 mg capsules
Take ONE capsule DAILY
Siobhan O'Toole

Today's date · Name of pharmacy and address

Keep out of reach and sight of children

28 Simvastatin 40 mg tablets
Take ONE tablet DAILY
Siobhan O'Toole

Today's date · Name of pharmacy and address

Pharmaceutical Care Plan	Name of student:

Date xx **Patient initials** SOT **DOB** 01/04/75 **Hospital number** 010203 **Gender** Female	**Date admitted** xx	**Tick sources used for medication history**

Allergies/Drug sensitivities

Allergen/drug (generic name)	Type of reaction (e.g. rash)
....	....
....	....
....	....
....	....
Signature:	Date: ....

No known allergies

Signature: .... Date: ....

Past medical history: Hypothyroidism Depression Hypercholester-olaemia	Patient Patient Relative/carer GP surgery GP letter GP repeat list Emergency Care Summary Community Pharmacy Patients Own Drugs Patient medication list Medical notes Nursing/residential home list Recent discharge prescription Other: .....

Presenting complaint(s): Suspected DVT

Diagnosis: DVT

Medication history confirmed (sign and date): ....

Medicines *prior* to admission

Medicine name, strength, form and route	Dose and frequency

	GP details	Community pharmacy details	Height* (m) .... Weight (kg) 60kgs
name	**Not required**	**Not required**	**BMI*** (weight[kg]/height [m²]): **not required**
address			Underweight <18.5
			Ideal 18.5–25
			Overweight 25–30
tel. number			Obese >30

Figure 4.6 Partially completed pharmaceutical care plan for Siobhan O'Toole.

OSCE Candidate notes page (for OSCE 4.1)

Candidate name:		Date:	

You may use the space below to make notes before speaking with the patient.
You will submit this page however it will **not** be assessed.

OSCE medication history – Script for patient actor (for OSCE 4.1)

You are Mrs Siobhan O'Toole, a 39-year-old woman who has been admitted to Medical Admissions Unit via A&E with a suspected deep vein thrombosis (DVT). Your husband took you to A&E the previous night, after you complained of a painful right leg which was red, swollen and tender.

You suffer from an underactive thyroid (*hypothyroidism*), for which you take *levothyroxine 50 μg daily*. You also have iron deficiency anaemia, for which you take *ferrous fumarate 305 mg daily*. You had your appendix removed when you were six.

The only medicine that you buy (without a prescription) is St. John's Wort (1 daily) for *low mood*. You get this from the local herbal shop.

You've brought your medicine boxes in with you, which you grabbed from the kitchen cupboard when leaving to go to hospital. You were due to obtain a new supply today. **This bag also includes your husband's levothyroxine, which you lifted by mistake instead of yours.**

The candidates need to ask to see your own medicines within the first three minutes.

If they do not do this within the first three minutes, you should then present the candidate with the medicines you have brought with you (but they will lose marks).

You must not tell the candidate that the levothyroxine belongs to your husband, unless probed.

Problems with patient's own medicines:

- Will include your husband's levothyroxine instead of yours – he will be taking 100 μg daily.

- Will not include the St John's wort.

You are **allergic to penicillin** (severe rash, difficulty breathing).

You **do not smoke** and **drink one small glass of wine on a Saturday and Sunday night.**

In case asked, your date of birth is **01/04/75** and you weigh **60 kg.** Your address is **1 Lisnagrilly Hall, Portadown.**

OSCE medication history – Script for patient actor (for OSCE 4.1)

If the candidate does not identify you, say...

'Are you sure that you are talking to the right person? There are two Mrs O'Tooles on this ward'

If the candidate asks if you have any allergies, say...

'I am allergic to penicillin.' – Do not prompt them about this.

If the candidate asks about the nature of the allergy, say...

'I develop a severe rash and find difficulty breathing.' – Do not prompt them about this.

If the candidate asks what medicines you take, say...

'I cannot remember their names, one for the thyroid, one for anaemia, and one to help mood.'

If the candidate asks you if you have brought any of your medicines in or a list, say...

'Yes – I brought my medicines with me.' (*Give candidates the bag of medicines*)' – Do not give them this unless they ask for it or 3 minutes have elapsed (whichever is sooner).

If asked, you can tell the candidate the *names only* of the medicines below. If they prompt/ask you also about doses and indication (what the medicine is being taken for) you can provide the other information provided below...

Drug Name	Dose/frequency	Indication	In POD bag?
Levothyroxine	50 µg daily	Thyroid gland removed – to replace thyroid hormone.	Yes – but you have lifted your **husband's** levothyroxine by mistake
Simvastatin	40 mg nocte	Hypercholesterolaeamia	Yes
Ferrous fumarate	305 mg daily	Iron – for iron deficiency anaemia	Yes
St John's wort	1 daily	Low mood	No
No recent vaccines	No	N/A	No (candidate should ask about this)

If the candidate asks you if you buy any medicines from the chemist, or garage etc ('Over the counter' medicines), say...

'I buy St John's wort for low mood from the herbal shop – I take one tablet every day.' *(This will not be in POD bag.)*

If the candidate asks if you smoke or drink alcohol, say...

'I do not smoke but like a small glass of wine on a Saturday and Sunday night.'

If the candidate asks if you are concordant/adherent with your medicines, say...

'Yes, I never forget to take my medication.'

If the candidate asks if you get your medicines in monthly/weekly quantities, say...

'I get my medicines every month.'

If the candidate asks you if you have any questions you would like to ask, say...

'No thanks – I'm all questioned out!'

👥 Buddy activity

Example 4.2.   Third-Year OSCE Examination

Please read the following information carefully. You have 10 minutes to complete the activity.

Background

You are a pharmacist working on a medical ward.

Mr James Hewitt has been admitted with suspected heart failure.

Past medical/surgical history

Hypertension

Chronic obstructive pulmonary disease (COPD)

Hearing loss

Activity

1. Establish Mr Hewitt's medication history.

You are NOT required to decide if medicines should be stopped, withheld or started.

2. Document the medication history on the front page of the partially completed pharmaceutical care plan provided.

3. You are assessed on what you say to the patient, your communication style as well as what you document on the pharmaceutical care plan.

You are provided with sources for the medication history, including the patient.

There are two people seated at the station: the examiner and the patient. Introduce yourself to the patient when you are ready to begin.

Please submit your completed medication history to the examiner at the end of the OSCE and do not forget to include your name on the form.

DO NOT write on or remove any materials provided.

Station props that would be provided

Item required

1. Instructions for candidate.

2. Script for patient actor.

3. Candidate answer sheet.

4. GP medication list for Mr James Hewitt (Fig. 4.7).

5. Mark sheet.

6. BNF.

7. Page 1 of partially completed care plan for Mr James Hewitt (Fig. 4.8)

Ballyhackamore Surgery, Belfast

Dr Johnston
Ballyhackamore
Belfast

Mr James Hewitt
DOB: 3-4-1939
17, The Manse
Ballyhackamore
Belfast

1/07/16	Amlodipine 10 mg tablets. Take one tablet in the morning	X 28	repeat
1/07/16	Tiotropium HandiHaler 18 microgram. Inhale one dose in the morning	X 1	repeat
1/07/16	Salbutamol 100 microgram Evohaler. Inhale two puffs prn	X 1	repeat
1/07/16	Fluticasone 250 micrograms Evohaler. Inhale one puff twice daily	X 1	repeat

Allergies: Aspirin

Use this reminder when ordering your repeat prescriptions.

Figure 4.7 GP medication list.

Medicines Reconciliation Form	Name of student:

Date xxxxx Patient initials JH DOB 3-4-1939 Hospital number CAH12345 Gender M	Date admitted xxxxxxx	Tick sources used for medication history

Allergies/Drug sensitivities		Past medical history: Hypertension COPD Hearing loss	Patient Patient Relative/carer GP surgery GP letter GP repeat list Emergency Care Summary Electronic care record Community Pharmacy Patients Own Drugs Patient medication list Medical notes Nursing/residential home list Recent discharge prescription Other: .....
Allergen/drug (generic name) .... **Signature:**	Type of reaction (e.g. rash) .... **Date:**		
No known allergies **Signature:** .... **Date:**			

Presenting complaint(s): Increasing shortness of breath	**Medication history confirmed** (sign and date): ....
Diagnosis: suspected heart failure	

Medicines *prior* to admission

Medicine name, strength, form and route	Dose and frequency

	GP details	Community pharmacy details	Height* (m) .... Weight (kg)...........
name	Not required	Not required	BMI* (weight[kg]/height [m²]): **not required**
address	Not required	Not required	Underweight <18.5
			Ideal 18.5–25
			Overweight 25–30
tel. number	Not required	Not required	Obese >30

Figure 4.8 Partially completed care plan for Mr James Hewitt (for OSCE 4.2).

OSCE Candidate notes page (for OSCE 4.2)

Candidate name:		Date:	

You may use the space below to make notes before speaking with the patient.
You will submit this page however it **will not** be assessed.

OSCE medication history – Script for patient actor (for OSCE 4.2)—cont'd

If the candidate has not asked for your list after two minutes talking, say...

'Oh! I forgot, I brought in this list.'

Once the candidate has got the medicines from you, they should verbally confirm that you take the medicines as detailed below ...

Drug Name	Strength	Dose	Frequency	Form	Route	Indication	On list?
Amlodipine	10 mg	1	Morning	Tablet	Oral	Hypertension	Yes
Tiotropium	18 µg	1 dose	Morning	HandiHaler	Inhaled	COPD	Yes
Salbutamol	100 µg/inh	2 puffs	PRN	Evohaler	Inhaled	COPD	Yes
Fluticasone	250 µg	1 puff	Twice daily	Evohaler	Inhaled	COPD	Yes

If the candidate asks you if you buy any medicines from the chemist, or garage etc ('Over the counter' medicines), say...

'No, I've enough of them from the doctor.'

If the candidate asks you if you have had any vaccinations in the last year, say...

'Any what? Any jabs? Is that what you're asking? Do I? I got the flu jab in October, that's about it...'

If candidates asks if you smoke or drink alcohol, say...

'I used to but not anymore – not allowed to!'

Establishing concordance/adherence:

If candidates ask if you are concordant/adherent with your medicines (but do not use layman's terms), say...

'Do I what? I don't understand what you mean.'

If the candidate asks if you are concordant/adherent with your medicines (using layman's terms with the same meaning), say...

'Do I what? Do I take them? My medicines? I do, I take them all...'

Possible further questioning:

If the candidate asks how much you weigh, say...

'My weight? How heavy I am? I have no clue – I think the last time I weighed myself I was about 13 stone?...'

If the candidate asks if you get your medicines monthly/weekly quantities, say...

'I phone up every month and get what the Dr gives me...'

If the candidate asks if you look after your own medicines, say...

'I do indeed...with help from the wife...'

If the candidate asks you if you have any questions you would like to ask, say...

'No, nothing at all...'

If the candidate asks you anything that is not relevant to this activity say...

'I don't think that is relevant...'

Closure of conversation:

The candidate should close the consultation by thanking you for your time and saying goodbye plus or minus any further points for clarification.

Buddy activity

Example 4.3. Second-Year OSCE Examination

Please read the following information carefully. You have 10 minutes to complete the activity

Background

You are a pharmacist working on the Medical Admissions Unit

Miss Margaret Jones is a 70-year-old woman admitted following a fall.

Past medical/surgical history

Asthma

Activity

1. Establish Miss Margaret Jones's medication history.

2. Document the medication history on the front page of the partially completed pharmaceutical care plan provided.

You are provided with sources for the medication history, including the patient. There are two people seated at the station: the examiner and the patient. Introduce yourself to the patient when you are ready to begin.

Please submit your completed medication history to the examiner at the end of the OSCE and do not forget to include your name on the form.

DO NOT write on or remove any materials provided.

Station props that would be provided

Item required

1. Instructions for candidate.

2. Script for patient actor.

3. Candidate notes sheet.

4. Mark sheet.

5. BNF.

6. GP medication list for Miss Margaret Jones (Fig. 4.9).

7. Partially completed care plan for Miss Margaret Jones (Fig. 4.10).

CASTLELANE MEDICAL CENTRE
RANDALSTOWN

26.06.16

Patient Details   **DOB** 3.10.1944
Miss Margaret Jones
36 Upper Hill
Dunganon
County Tyrone

Current Medication

Budesonide 400 microgram Turbohaler	inhale two metered doses bd	last issued 26/02/2015	1 inhaler
Terbutaline 500 microgram Turbohaler	inhale one metered dose prn	last issued 26/02/2015	2 inhalers

Acutes
None issued within past 6 months

Drug Intolerances
None recorded

Figure 4.9 GP medication list.

Medicines Reconciliation Form	Name of student:
Document your answer to question 2 on this answer sheet.	

Date xxxx Patient initials MJ DOB 3/10/1944 Gender Female	Date admitted xxxxx	Tick sources used for medication history
Allergies/Drug sensitivities Allergen/drug (generic name) ⋮ Type of reaction (e.g. rash) Signature: ⋮ Date: **No known allergies** Signature: .... Date:	Past medical history: Asthma	Patient Patient Relative/carer GP surgery GP letter GP repeat list Emergency Care Summary Community Pharmacy Patients Own Drugs Patient medication list Medical notes Nursing/residential home list Recent discharge prescription Other: .....
Presenting complaint(s): Fall, ankle pain **Diagnosis:** sprained ankle	Medication history confirmed (sign and date):	

Medicines *prior* to admission

Medicine name, strength, form and route	Dose and frequency

	GP details	Community pharmacy details	Height* (m) .... Weight (kg)...........
name	Not required	Not required	BMI* (weight[kg]/height [m²]): **not required**
address			Underweight <18.5
			Ideal 18.5–25
			Overweight 25–30
tel. number			Obese >30

Figure 4.10 Partially completed care plan for Miss Margaret Jones (for OSCE 4.3).

OSCE Candidate notes page (for OSCE 4.3)

Candidate name:		Date:	

Use the space below to make any notes before you take the medication history.
This notes page is not assessed.

Example 4.3: Second-year OSCE station – Notes to patient actor

Background

Name: Miss Margaret Jones

Age: 70

DOB: 3.10.1944

Address: 36 Upper Hill, Dungannon

Weight: 56 kg

- The candidate MUST to ask to see your own medicines (PODs) or additional source such as list of medications etc.

- If the candidate does not ask you for the second source and tries to establish the medication history using you as the only source, act vague and see script below.

- Two minutes after the candidates have begun to speak if they still have not asked for your second source, suddenly 'remember' that you have the list and give it to the candidate (see script below). Candidate will lose a mark for this prompt.

- If the candidate does not begin to speak until the final 2 minutes of the allocated station time, give the source straight away. Candidate will lose a mark for this prompt.

OSCE medication history – Script for patient actor (for OSCE 4.3)

If the candidate does not identify you, say...

'Are you sure that you are talking to the right person? Just want to be sure it's me you want...'

If the candidate asks your date of birth, address or weight, say...

'My date of birth is 3.10.1944. My address is 36 Upper Hill, Dungannon, weight 56 kg

If the candidate asks what name you would like to be called say:

'Everybody calls me Peggy.'

If the candidate asks if you have any allergies, say...

'No, I'm not allergic to anything.' – Do not prompt the candidate about this.

If the candidate asks what medicines you take (but has not asked for your PODs or a written document at this stage) say...

'I take a puffer for my asthma every morning and night and I also have another that I take sometimes.'

If the candidate asks what the medicines are for, say...

'They are puffers for my breathing.'

If the candidate asks what strengths and doses you take, say...

'Can you help me?'

If the candidate asks you if you have brought any PODs in, say...

'No, I never thought to' or something to this effect.

If the candidate asks you if you have brought in a written list of medicines (or other form of document), say...

'Yes, here it is.'

If the candidate has not asked for your list/PODs after two minutes talking, say...

'Oh! I forgot, I brought in this list.'

OSCE medication history – Script for patient actor (for OSCE 4.3)—cont'd

Drug Name	Strength	Dose	Frequency	Form	Route	Indication (FOR INFO ONLY)	On list/ present?
Budesonide	400 µg	Two puffs	BD	Turbohaler	Inhaled	Asthma	Yes
Terbutaline	500 µg	One puff	PRN	Turbohaler	Inhaled	Asthma	Yes
Paracetamol	500 mg	1g	4 hourly PRN	Tablet	Oral	Headache	No – only volunteer if asked

If the candidate asks you if you buy any medicines from the chemist, or garage etc ('Over the counter' medicines), say...

'No – oh I do get painkillers the odd time for a headache. If they prompt you more... 'Paracetamol.' If they prompt you more about dose and frequency, 'I take two tablets when I get a sore head. The pharmacist said I should take no more than eight in a day and leave four hours between doses.'

If the candidate asks if you smoke or drink alcohol, say...

'I don't take any alcohol and I don't smoke.'

If the candidate asks if you are concordant/adherent with your medicines (or uses layman's terms with the same meaning), say...

'I always take them the way the doctor tells me to.'

If the candidate asks if you get your medicines monthly/weekly quantities, say...

'I get them monthly usually.'

If the candidate asks if you look after your own medicines, say...

'Yes.'

If the candidate asks you if you have had any vaccinations in the last year, say...

'No.'

If the candidate asks you if you have any questions you would like to ask, say...

'No that's fine.'

If the candidate asks if there is anything else he/she can do for you, say...

'No thanks.'

If the candidate asks you anything that is not relevant to this activity say...

'I don't think that is relevant...'

The candidate should close the consultation by thanking you for your time and saying goodbye plus or minus any further points for clarification.

OSCE medication history – Mark sheet (for OSCE 4.1)

Candidate's Name		Date	

Assessment Criteria for Example 4.1:	Mark		
Communication points			
1. Introduces themselves including name **(1 mark)** and position **(1 mark)**	0	1	2
2. Identifies this is correct patient using name and one other unique identifier	0	1	–
3. Explains the purpose of the discussion i.e. ascertaining medicines patient uses at home. *Terms such as 'wee chat' or 'just wanted to talk to you about your medicines' do not achieve a mark.*	0	1	–
4. Fully documents the patient has an allergy to penicillin **(1)** and that it causes rash and difficulty breathing **(1)**	0	1	2
5. Verifies all medicines verbally (including vaccines) **(2 marks)**, some medicines **(1 mark)**	0	1	2

Prompt to obtain second source for medication history

6. Subtract one mark if actor has to prompt candidate to obtain PODs	–1

Documents each medicine name **(1 mark)**, strength **(1 mark)**, number of dose units **(1 mark)**, frequency **(1 mark)**, route **(1 mark)** and dosage form **(1 mark)** on the care plan (including vaccines if appropriate).
Criteria in **bold italics** are essential i.e. *name, strength, dose, frequency*.

7. ***Levothyroxine: 50 µg; tablet: one** tablet **once daily** oral*	0	1	2	3	4	5	6
8. ***Ferrous fumarate: 305 mg:** inhaler: **one** tablet **once daily:** oral*	0	1	2	3	4	5	6
9. ***St John's Wort: one tablet once daily:** oral*	0	1	2	3	4	5	6
10. ***Simvastatin: 40 mg: one** tablet **once at night:** oral*	0	1	2	3	4	5	6

11. Documents the following on the pharmaceutical care plan. Sources acknowledged:		
a. Patient	0	1
b. PODs	0	1
c. Signs that drug history confirmed	0	1
12. Thanks the patient for time/help	0	1
13. Asks patient if he or she has any questions	0	1

DiscretionaryAny other valid point (only awarded if full marks not obtained elsewhere)

14. Any other valid point up to a maximum of 2 points	0	1	2
• Lifestyle advice			
• Other _____			

Continued

95

OSCE Mark sheet (for OSCE 4.2)—cont'd

Professionalism including communication style

Excellent	**All of the time:** appropriately attentive: empathetic and interested: identifies and resolves health promotion issues: doesn't cause embarrassment or loss of face: checks understanding: organised questioning: body language appropriate & eye contact good.	4
Good	**Most of the time (as above).**	3
Average	**Some of the time (as above).**	2
Poor	**Most of the time:** inattentive: lack of empathy and interest: does not identify or resolve health promotion issues: causes embarrassment or loss of face: does not check understanding: disorganised questioning: body language inappropriate & eye contact poor.	1
Fail	**All of the time (as above).**	0

If candidates propose any course of action which could lead to serious harm or death, they will **fail** the OSCE. Always seek a second opinion. Give detail: _____

Total Mark:		/44	
Angoff 25 Criteria in bold italics are essential (aspects of 7–10).		**Pass**	**Fail**

Assessor's comments:

Assessor's Signature:_____

OSCE Mark sheet (for OSCE 4.3)

Candidate's Name		Date	

Communication points

1. Introduce themselves including name **(1 mark)** and position **(1 mark)**	0	1	2
2. Identifies that this is the correct patient using name and one other unique identifier	0	1	–
3. Explains the purpose of the discussion i.e. ascertaining medicines patient uses at home. Terms such as 'wee chat' or 'just want to talk to you about your medicines' do not score.	0	1	–
4. Fully documents the patient has no known drug allergies	0	1	–
5. Verifies all medicines verbally (including vaccines) **(2 marks)**, some medicines **(1 mark)**	0	1	2
6. Subtract one mark if actor has to prompt candidate to obtain GP list	–1		

Documents each medicine name **(1 mark)**, strength **(1 mark)**, form **(1 mark)**, route **(1 mark)**, dose **(1 mark)** and frequency **(1 mark)** on the care plan

7. Budesonide 400 µg Turbohaler, inhaled, two puffs/inhalations/metered doses, twice daily	0	1	2	3	4	5	6
8. Terbutaline 500 µg Turbohaler, inhaled, one puff/inhalation/metered dose, PRN	0	1	2	3	4	5	6
9. Paracetamol 500 mg tablet, oral, 1 g (or two tablets), every four hours (or 4–6 hourly) up to eight a day PRN	0	1	2	3	4	5	6

10. **Documents** sources acknowledged on the pharmaceutical care plan:		
• Patient	0	1
• GP repeat list	0	1
• Sign and date that history is confirmed	0	1
11. Asks patient if he has any questions	0	1
12. Thanks the patient/closes the conversation appropriately	0	1

Knowledge points

13. Establishes patient has no known drug allergies	0	1
14. Award 1 mark for any other valid point, for example:		
• Smoking status, alcohol consumption, concordance	0	1

Professionalism including communication style

Excellent	**All of the time:** appropriately attentive with patient: empathetic and interested: identifies and resolves problems e.g. if patient drinks or smokes attempted health promotion: doesn't cause embarrassment or loss of face to patient: checks patient understanding by asking patient to repeat back (counselling) or repeating back (history taking), organised questioning/provision of information: body language appropriate & eye contact good.	4

Continued

OSCE Mark sheet (for OSCE 4.3)—cont'd

Good	Most of the time (as above).	3
Average	Some of the time (as above).	2
Poor	**Most of the time:** inattentive with patient: lack of empathy and interest: lack of problem identification or resolution: causes embarrassment or loss of face to patient: omitted check of patient understanding by asking patient to repeat back (counselling) or repeating back (history taking), disorganised questioning/provision of information: body language inappropriate, eye contact poor.	1
Fail	All of the time (as above).	0

If candidates propose any course of action which could lead to serious harm, they will **fail** the OSCE. Always seek a second opinion. Give detail: _____

Total Mark:	/36	
Angoff score (borderline competence): 21	**Pass**	**Fail**

Assessor's comments:

Assessor's Signature:_____

✔ How to excel in this type of station

Action	Reason	How
Be systematic	To ensure you don't miss anything and to maintain patient safety, follow your medication history procedure including using at least 2 sources for your medication history.	Ideally, obtain a list of the patient's medication or the actual medication boxes and tablets from the patient or carer who is present at the station. Confirm the details on the list with the patient or carer. Enquire about adherence to the prescribed doses and times of administration as these may differ from those prescribed and may affect medication effectiveness.
Check about non-prescribed medicines use	Patient safety; you need to ensure that the patient is not buying something unsuitable in the supermarket or the pharmacy or using their partners medication inappropriately.	When you have confirmed the patient's prescribed medications and doses, ask about other medicines purchased or used. You will need to confirm the doses, frequency and the reasons for use with the patient. You may uncover use of inappropriate medications e.g. use of husband's pain killers or purchase of over the counter pseudoephedrine in a patient with hypertension and you will need to address this with your patient.
Confirm the final list with the patient / carer	You have asked a lot of information and have recorded this on the Pharmaceutical Care Plan form or equivalent (e.g. Medicines Reconciliation form). Take time to confirm this final list with the patient or carer prior to advising this for prescribing on the medication chart.	Read out the final list to the patient / carer and ask them after each medication if this is right. This is a good way of self-checking your final list prior to the patient being prescribed the medication.
Balance your time between speaking to the patient and writing your information on the Med Rec form	Some students spend a long time talking to their patient and don't leave enough time to record their information on the Medicines Reconciliation form or make errors by rushing the recording of the information.	If you do not record the information or record it inaccurately you will put the patient at risk.

✗ Common errors in this type of station

Action	Remedy	Reason
Missing medications from the final list	Remember to ask about all medications that the patient takes on a regular basis including those which have been purchased from the pharmacy or supermarket. It is also vital to ask about medicines which the patient may receive directly from the hospital e.g. intravenous antibiotics or high cost items. Confirming the final list you have recorded with the patient is an excellent way of second checking your information prior to its prescription.	If you miss a medication off the final list, the patient will not receive it during their inpatient stay and it may compromise their improvement. It is possible that if the medicine is omitted that another similar medicine is prescribed during the admission and may lead to therapeutic duplication on discharge and potential restarting of the original medication. It is also possible that on discharge the omission of a medication could lead the GP will think this medication has been deliberately omitted from the patient's list and they may stop it erroneously.
Transcription errors with unfamiliar medications.	If you are transcribing medicines with which you are unfamiliar e.g. with doses or frequencies, you may make an error in the recording of their details. Always check unfamiliar medications in the BNF. Errors in the recording of micrograms as milligrams are also common.	An error in transcription can lead to the patient receiving an under or over dose.
Not recording the purchased over counter medications on the medicines reconciliation form	Although you have asked the patient about their over the counter medication use, it is vital that you record this information on the medicines reconciliation form; including the dose and frequency of use.	If this information is not recorded, the medical team will not be aware that this medicine is in regular use and it can lead to therapeutic duplication or drug-drug interactions.

Further reading

Bajcar, J., 2006. Activity analysis of patients' medication-taking practice and the role of making sense: A grounded theory study. Res. Social Adm. Pharm. 2 (1), 59–82.

Cornish, P.L., Knowles, S.R., Marcheso, R., et al., 2005. Unintended medication discrepancies at the time of hospital admission. Arch. Intern. Med. 165, 424–429.

Karnon, J., Campbell, F., Czoski-Murray, C., 2009. Model-based cost-effectiveness analysis of interventions aimed at preventing medication error at hospital admission (medicines reconciliation). J. Eval. Clin. Pract. 15 (2), 299–306(8).

Vira, T., Colquhoun, M., Etchells, E.E., 2006. Reconcilable differences: correcting medication errors at hospital admission and discharge. Qual. Saf. Health Care 15 (2), 122–126.

Introduction

Medicines Optimisation is a term which refers to the desire to maximise the beneficial clinical outcomes for patients from their prescribed and purchased medicines with an emphasis on patient safety as well as professional and patient collaboration. It places patients at the centre of their healthcare, taking a holistic approach built on partnerships between clinical professionals and the patients they care for. The management of complex conditions is shifting more and more from hospital to primary care, reinforcing the importance of medicines optimisation across all sectors of pharmacy.

The main difference in relation to 'pharmaceutical care' is that pharmaceutical care can be defined as:

> *'The responsible provision of drug therapy for the purpose of achieving definite outcomes that improve a patient's quality of life.'* – (Hepler & Strand, 1990).

Pharmaceutical care in the United Kingdom has evolved from the pharmacist's role as a healthcare practitioner in the community, particularly within community pharmacies. Community pharmacists have always provided medication for patients on an individual basis and offered advice to meet patient needs. Over the past 25 years the advisory role of the pharmacist has developed in all sectors of healthcare particularly as the boundaries between healthcare sectors become increasingly blurred and sicker patients are discharged for community healthcare management (TYC, 2011). *Clinical Pharmacy* is now used to illustrate the knowledge, skills and behaviours required by a pharmacist who will contribute to patient care. It has become an essential aspect of the patient's management both in community, hospital and intermediate healthcare settings.

There are three key aspects of pharmaceutical care which help to describe what pharmacists and pharmacy students providing pharmaceutical care should strive to achieve:

1. *The responsible provision of drug therapy*

Pharmacists share responsibility for the consequences of medication use in and by patients. The pharmacist has a legal responsibility to protect the patient from demonstrable harm, for example an adverse drug reaction or an incorrectly dispensed item. Pharmacists also have a moral responsibility to protect the patient from suboptimal drug therapy through their professional activity, for example an underdose in a paediatric patient due to incorrect weight calculation.

2. *Definite (patient) outcomes*

In order to protect patients against suboptimal treatment, healthcare professionals must work in tandem to develop and manage desired patient outcomes. Strong teamwork between all staff managing the patient enables pharmacists to align their professional objectives in accordance with patients' needs. A key aspect of a pharmacist's role in patient management is the determination of the exact purpose of drug treatment and any risks associated with its use (*problem or risk*) as well as the desired patient outcomes both **before** and **during** the provision of drug therapy (*goals of therapy*) and how these will be achieved (*action*). Pharmaceutical care is usually delivered over a period of time and by a number of team members and so it makes sense that this work is documented to support ongoing therapeutic decisions (*pharmaceutical care plan*).

As a suggested template for a pharmaceutical care plan (see Table 5.1 below), we have developed this system outline above. During this chapter, we will revisit this format to illustrate the development and recording of pharmaceutical care for individual patients.

Table 5.1		
Pharmaceutical care issue or risk	**Therapeutic goal**	**Action(s)**
	What is the ideal outcome for your patient?	*Action(s) you would take as a pharmacist to reach this goal in your patient*

3. *Quality of life*

When developing patient goals, it is important that you consider the impact on your individual patient's quality of life, for example do not recommend that a patient conducts aerobic exercise for 30 minutes up to five times per week if he or she has just experienced a disabling ischaemic stroke. Develop achievable goals for your individual patients taking into consideration their own personal goals and lifestyle.

Pharmaceutical care issues

The provision of pharmaceutical care includes the identification, prevention and resolution of medication-related problems or *pharmaceutical care issues* (PCIs). PCIs can be described as risks identified in the therapeutic management plan for an individual patient which actually or potentially interferes with desirable health outcomes. The most common PCIs are the identification and resolution of adverse drug reactions and interactions, inappropriate drug selection based on individual patient characteristics, inappropriate dosing, and inappropriate drug use or administration.

There are a number of ways in which you can improve a patient's quality of life by identifying PCIs and they are practised in every sector of pharmacy. We have divided these up into a number of approaches to help you to identify the key aspects. These are the types of competencies which may be included in Medicines Optimisation OSCEs; they will vary depending on the topic and task required in the OSCE time period (see Table 5.2).

Table 5.2 GPhC Competencies assessed by this type of OSCE station		Third year	Fourth year
10.2.1 (b)	access and critically evaluate evidence to support safe, rational and cost-effective use of medicines	*shows how*	*shows how*
10.2.1 (h)	Provide evidence-based medicines information	*shows how*	*shows how*
10.2.2 (c)	Instruct patients in the safe and effective use of their medicines and devices	*shows how*	*shows how*

Table 5.2   GPhC Competencies assessed by this type of OSCE station—cont'd

		Third year	Fourth year
10.2.2 (f)	provide, monitor and modify prescribed treatment to maximise health outcomes	shows how	shows how
10.2.2 (g)	Communicate with patients about their prescribed treatment	shows how	shows how
10.2.2 (h)	optimise treatment for individual patient needs in collaboration with the prescriber	shows how	shows how
10.2.3 (c)	use pharmaceutical calculations to verify the safety of doses and administration rates	shows how	shows how
10.2.4 (h)	Provide accurate written or oral information appropriate to the needs of patients, the public or other healthcare professionals	shows how	shows how
10.2.5 (a)	Demonstrate the characteristics of a prospective professional pharmacist as set out in relevant codes of conduct and behaviour	Does	Does

How to … clinically screen medications on a hospital inpatient's medication kardex or medication chart

When you are undertaking a review of a ward of patients, you often start your patient review by reviewing the patient's inpatient medication kardex/chart. The review or 'clinical screen' of medications should be approached in a stepwise fashion to ensure each medication is safe and suitable for each patient. Remember that each patient is an individual with specific requirements: consider the reason for admission, diagnoses, key signs/symptoms and their bearing on the prescription you are reviewing. You should make use of the patient multi-professional notes and all other monitoring charts at the patient bedside.

There isn't always a clear-cut solution, and therefore a pharmacist's clinical judgement should always be used. When a number of options exist, they may need to be weighed on a risk-benefit basis so as to decide on the most appropriate plan of action.

Stepwise approach to screening (questions to ask yourself)

1. Check and confirm patient allergy status before continuing
2. Is there an indication for the medication, why is it prescribed? Is it contraindicated? Is there therapeutic duplication?
3. Is the dose and frequency suitable and safe for the patient?
4. Is the current dosage form the most suitable for the patient?
5. Are any of the above affected by the patient's current condition?
6. Are any of the above affected by clinical findings (blood pressure [BP], heart rate) or laboratory tests (renal function/creatinine clearance, sodium or potassium levels, liver function tests, full blood count)? E.g. if BP is low, should you recommend holding an antihypertensive? If heart rate (HR) is low, should you recommend holding a beta blocker? If temperature is raised, is the patient on an antipyretic?

If eGFR (estimated Glomerular Filtration Rate) is decreased, you need to check appropriateness of medication and doses. If potassium is high, could any of the medicines be contributing to this? Etc.

7. Is the medication considered 'high risk' or a 'trigger' drug i.e. requiring more thorough consideration e.g. due to a narrow therapeutic index (digoxin, warfarin), high risk of adverse effects (methotrexate, amiodarone) or interactions (simvastatin, clarithromycin), etc.?
8. Does the medication interact with other medications, food or disease states?
9. Is the prescribing both legible (clearly written) and legal (signature, dose, start date etc. present)?

Example 1

Mr SP, an 78-year-old male, admitted with an ischaemic stroke, is 'nil by mouth' and therefore cannot take oral medications at present (due to risk of aspiration). He has no known drug allergies. He is on digoxin.

Reviewing the kardex for Mr SP in Figure 5.1, what are the 'pharmaceutical care issues' that need to be considered?

(*Suggested answers are provided that you may find in a patient's case notes*).

These questions represent the issues you should consider as you review the medication kardex and case notes for PCIs in your patient in relation to digoxin:

1. Why is Mr SP taking digoxin? What is the indication, is it listed?
   a. Yes it is listed, the case notes show a past medical history (PMHx) of heart failure
      i. It can also be used for Atrial fibrillation (AF) – what else would you need prescribed for your patient if this was the case?
      ii. Bearing in mind your patient has had an ischaemic stroke, would you alter any of this other medication? E.g. Does he require anticoagulant therapy? have you completed a CHADsVASc and HASBLED for him?
   b. Some stroke patients may not be able to provide an oral history on admission and this information may have to be gleaned from previous admissions/relatives/GP.
2. Is the dose and frequency of administration suitable for Mr SP (in relation to the reason for prescription, his renal function, any co-morbid conditions or co-prescribed medications)?
   a. Unable to answer at this point, not all investigations are complete.
3. Is the dosage form (tablet) suitable for Mr SP given his reason for admission?
   a. No, the enteral (oral) route is not suitable, IV route is the only option (refer to the BNF for details)
4. Are there any issues switching between oral and IV (e.g. in relation to bioavailability and administration)?
   a. With digoxin, there are considerations (consult www.medicines.org.uk for conversion doses and administration information).
5. Will any of the clinical investigations/examinations affect the dose/administration of digoxin?
   a. Yes, BP, HR, respiratory rate should be checked pre- and postadministration of digoxin, especially HR. Digoxin administration should be discussed with the Multidisciplinary team (MDT) if Heart Rate (HR) <60 bpm.
   b. Serum K and renal function should be checked to ensure the patient is safe from adverse effects of digoxin.

Text continued on p. 112

WQA7000 Rev. October 2011

Medicine Prescription and Administration Record

Rewritten on (date): _____

Record: _/_ of _/_

Allergies / Medicine Sensitivities

THIS SECTION **MUST** BE COMPLETED

Date	Medicine (generic) / Allergen	Type of Reaction	Signature

OR

No Known allergies ☑ Please tick

Signature: *Dr Nairan* Date: 1.12.14

Admission Medicines Reconciliation completed

Sign: *E. Vernon* Date: 1.12.14

Discharge prescription ordered by

Sign: _____ Date: _____

Write in CAPITAL LETTERS or use addressograph

Surname: *P*

First Names: *S*

Hospital No: *W123456*

DOB: *10-11-36* Check identity

Hospital: *Altnagelvin* Ward: *Medical*

Consultant: *Dr. Jameson*

Date of Admission: *1.12.14*

Weight (Kg)	Date	Height (cm)
82	1-12-2014	185

Requirements for Prescribing and Administration

- Nurses must not administer medicines that are improperly or illegibly prescribed.
- Do not prescribe or administer medication if the allergy status is not documented and signed (unless in an emergency).
- Prescribe generically (refer to WHSCT Policy for appropriate use of approved/generic names of medicines).
- Print the full name of the medicine in CAPITALS in black ink. Do not abbreviate medicine names.
- Do not alter existing instructions. Cancel and rewrite any changes in medicine therapy.
- Discontinue any therapy by drawing a diagonal line through the prescription and the remainder of the administration record. Enter the date of discontinuation and signature in the 'Stop' space.
- Do not abbreviate 'micrograms', 'nanograms', 'international units' or units; write in full.
- Prescriber's signatures must be written in full; initials are not acceptable.
- Other prescriptions in use must be referenced on the main prescription record.
- Attach all additional charts to the Medicine Prescription and Administration record.
- The administering nurse(s) must initial each administration.
- All kardexes must be rewritten after 14 days.
- Medicines reconciliation - for each regular or when required medicine, indicate changes made to therapy during stay.
    - On admission, refer to the patient's documented medication history, reconcile medicines on the kardex and circle 'no change', 'increased dose', 'decreased dose' or 'new' medicine accordingly.
    - During patient stay, ensure any subsequent changes are similarly indicated and document the reason in the table below.
    - At discharge, ensure information on medicine changes (including stopped medication) is sent to the GP.

Additional Charts in Use (please tick)

Epidural ☐	Intrathecal ☐	Blood Sugar Monitoring ☐	Total Parenteral Nutrition (TPN) ☐	Other (please specify) ☐
Patient Controlled Analgesia ☐	Diabetic Ketoacidosis ☐	Fluid Balance ☐	Oral Anticoagulant ☑	Syringe Driver (please indicate 1 or more) ☐
Insulin ☐	Chemotherapy ☐	Anaesthetic Record ☐	Endoscopy ☐	

Special Instructions / Additional Notes on Medicines / Reason for Medicine Omission (please sign and date)

Medicines Reconciliation Record During Patient's Stay

	Medication	Commenced in Hospital (tick if YES)	Stopped in Hospital (tick if YES)	Dose Changed ↑ or ↓	Reason for Medication Change
1					
2					
3					
4					
5					

OS17629

Figure 5.1 Medication kardex for Mr SP.

Continued

Venous Thromboembolism (VTE) Risk Assessment for Hospitalised Adults

Risk assessment must be completed on admission

Write in CAPITAL LETTERS or use addressograph

Surname: ___

First Names: ___

Hospital No: W123456

DOB: 10-11-1936 *check identity*

Step 1: Assess for level of mobility – All Patients

	Tick		Tick		Tick
Surgical patient		Medical patient expected to have ongoing reduced mobility relative to normal state	✓	Medical patient NOT expected to have significantly reduced mobility relative to normal state	
Assess for thrombosis and bleeding risk below (Complete steps 2 – 5)				Risk assessment complete (Go to step 5)	

Step 2: Review thrombosis risk

Any tick for thrombosis risk factors should prompt consideration for thromboprophylaxis

Patient related	Tick	Admission related	Tick
Active cancer or cancer treatment		Significantly reduced mobility for 3 days or more	✓
Age >60	✓	Hip or knee replacement	
Dehydration		Hip fracture	
Known thrombophilias		Total anaesthetic + surgery time > 90 minutes	
Personal history / first degree relative with history of VTE	.	Surgery involving pelvis or lower limb with anaesthetic + surgery time > 60 minutes	
One or more significant medical comorbidities (eg heart disease; metabolic, endocrine or respiratory pathologies; acute infectious diseases; inflammatory conditions)	✓	Acute surgical admission with inflammatory or intra-abdominal condition	
Obesity (BMI>30kg/m²)		Critical care admission	
Use of hormone replacement therapy		Surgery with significant reduction in mobility	
Use of oestrogen-containing oral contraceptive therapy		**The above risk factors are not exhaustive, additional risks may be considered. Other:**	
Varicose veins with phlebitis			
Pregnancy or < 6 weeks post partum (see obstetric risk assessment for VTE)			

Step 3: Review bleeding risk

Any tick should prompt staff to consider if bleeding risk is sufficient to preclude pharmacological intervention

Patient related	Tick	Admission related	Tick
Active bleeding		Neurosurgery, spinal surgery or eye surgery	
Acquired bleeding disorder (such as acute liver failure)		Lumbar puncture / epidural / spinal anaesthesia expected in the next 12 hours	
Concurrent use of anticoagulants known to increase risk of bleeding (such as warfarin with INR >2)		Lumbar puncture / epidural / spinal anaesthesia within the previous 4 hours	
Acute stroke		Other procedure with high bleeding risk	
Thrombocytopaenia (Platelets <75x10⁹/l)		**The above risk factors are not exhaustive, additional risks may be considered. Other:**	
Uncontrolled systolic hypertension (>230/120)			
Untreated inherited bleeding disorder (such as haemophilia and von Willebrand's disease)			

Step 4: Tick the appropriate risk category

Risk of VTE (tick)	High risk of VTE with low bleeding risk		High risk of VTE with significant bleeding risk		Low risk of VTE	✓
Thromboprophylaxis prescribed on kardex? (tick)	Yes	✓	Type Prescribed (tick)	Pharmacological e.g. LMWH		✓
	No			Mechanical		

Step 5: Signature

VTE risk assessed on admission	Signature: Dr Nave Print Name: J. NOVRAN Date and Time: 1.2.14 10am

VTE risk should be re-assessed within 24 hours and whenever clinical condition changes

Northern Ireland VTE Advisory Group, June 2011

2

Figure 5.1—cont'd

Regular Non-Injectable Medication
Check allergy status and patient identity

Codes for recording omitted doses

Ⓝ = nil by mouth Ⓥ = vomiting
Ⓡ = patient refused Ⓓ = drug not available
Ⓟ = patient not available Ⓞ = other*
Ⓢ = unable to swallow ⓄR = Prescribed omission*

*Record reasons in medical/nursing notes.

Take action on omitted doses as appropriate

Write in CAPITAL LETTERS or use addressograph

Surname: .....P.
First Names: .....S
Consultant: .....Dr. James Ward: Medical
Hospital No: W123456
D.O.B.: .....10-11-1936 Check identity

Year: 2014		Day and Month: →			½2	²/12	³/12	⁴/12								
Circle times or enter variable dose/time				▼ ▼												
Medicine Digoxin				06⁰⁰												
Dose 125 micrograms	Route 0	Start Date 1/12/14	Stop Date	08⁰⁰	✓	SP										
Special Instructions / Directions		Signature		12⁰⁰												
Medicines Reconciliation (circle)				14⁰⁰												
(No Change) Increased Dose · Decreased Dose · New				18⁰⁰												
Signature ⅂Novran Print Name J Novran Bleep 4669			Pharmacy	22⁰⁰												
Medicine Bisoprolol				06⁰⁰												
Dose 10 mg	Route 0	Start Date 1/12/14	Stop Date	08⁰⁰	✓	SP										
Special Instructions / Directions		Signature		12⁰⁰												
Medicines Reconciliation (circle)				14⁰⁰												
(No Change) Increased Dose · Decreased Dose · New				18⁰⁰												
Signature ⅂Novran Print Name J Novran Bleep 4669			Pharmacy SP	22⁰⁰												
Medicine Atorvastatin				06⁰⁰												
Dose 20 mg	Route 0	Start Date 1/12/14	Stop Date	08⁰⁰	✓	SP										
Special Instructions / Directions		Signature		12⁰⁰												
Medicines Reconciliation (circle)				14⁰⁰												
(No Change) Increased Dose · Decreased Dose · New				18⁰⁰												
Signature ⅂Novran Print Name J Novran Bleep 4669			Pharmacy	22⁰⁰												
Medicine Ramipril				06⁰⁰												
Dose 5 mg	Route 0	Start Date 1/12/14	Stop Date	08⁰⁰	✓	SP										
Special Instructions / Directions		Signature		12⁰⁰												
Medicines Reconciliation (circle)				14⁰⁰												
(No Change) Increased Dose · Decreased Dose · New				18⁰⁰												
Signature ⅂Novran Print Name J Novran Bleep 4669			Pharmacy	22⁰⁰												
Medicine Aspirin				06⁰⁰												
Dose 75 mg	Route 0	Start Date 1/12/14	Stop Date 1/12/14	08⁰⁰	✓	ⓄR										
Special Instructions / Directions		Signature S.Jam		12⁰⁰												
Medicines Reconciliation (circle)				14⁰⁰												
(No Change) Increased Dose · Decreased Dose · New				18⁰⁰												
Signature ⅂Novran Print Name Bleep 4669			Pharmacy	22⁰⁰												

Figure 5.1—cont'd

Continued

Once Only Medicines and Pre-Medications
(includes administration under Patient Group Direction)

If more than one Kardex, ensure 'once only' medicines are written on
'1 of 2' Kardex, until once only section on that Kardex is complete.

Patient Name: S. P.

Hospital Number: N123456
(complete if photocopying page)

Prescription						Administration		
Date	Medicine	Dose	Route	Time to be given (24 hour clock)	Signature	Given by	Time given (24 hour clock)	Pharmacy
1/12/14	ASPIRIN	300mg	O	8am	JNawe	SP.	8.15am	EV.

Figure 5.1—cont'd

As Required Medicines
Check for allergies / medicine sensitivities

Codes for recording omitted doses

(N) = nil by mouth	(V) = vomiting
(R) = patient refused	(D) = drug not available
(P) = patient not available	(O) = other*
(S) = unable to swallow	(OR) = Prescribed omission*

*Record reasons in medical/nursing notes.

Take action on omitted doses as appropriate

Write in CAPITAL LETTERS or use addressograph

Surname: P
First Names: S
Consultant: JAMESON Ward: Medical
Hospital No: H123456
D.O.B: 10-11-1936 Check identity

Medicine			Start Date	Date											
PARACETAMOL			1-12-14												
Dose 1g	Route O	Freq.(max) 4-6hrly	Stop Date	Time											
Special Instructions/Directions *max: 8 daily*				Signature											
				Dose/Route											
Signature J.Nouran		Bleep 4669		Pharmacy											
Print name J.NOURAN				Given By											
Medicine SENNA			Start Date	Date											
Dose 7.5mg	Route O	Freq.(max) 8hrly	Stop Date	Time											
Special Instructions/Directions				Signature											
				Dose/Route											
Signature JN		Bleep 4669		Pharmacy											
Print name J.NOURAN				Given By											

Figure 5.1—cont'd

6. Is digoxin considered 'high risk'?
   a. Yes, digoxin is a high risk drug, it has a narrow therapeutic index – considering Mr SP's acute condition, it would be appropriate to check a digoxin level.
   b. Remember that the level should be taken at steady state (5 × elimination half-life) and also 5–6 hours post oral dose, so if it is given at 8 am, level can be taken at 2 pm.
7. Does the medication interact with other medication, food or disease state?
   a. Check for clinically relevant interactions.
8. Should the digoxin dose be administered or would you advise holding it until more information has been gathered?
   a. This patient could be at risk of acute heart failure if digoxin is held, or of arrhythmias which may cause another cardiovascular event.
   b. Discuss with Multi-Disciplinary Team (MDT) if any other issues present, otherwise administer.

Using the same scenario for a non–high risk medication e.g. mebeverine (for irritable bowel syndrome), many of the steps would not be considered because it is not a 'high risk' drug etc hence there would be negligible risk posed to patients in withholding mebeverine while they were 'nil by mouth'.

Discharge

The patient's medication kardex is usually viewed during the patient's admission to secondary care, and a final check of the patients' medicines occurs when they are going home, when the discharge medications are reviewed. In this case you will have both the discharge prescription and the medication kardex to review together so that both issues of transcription (accuracy check) and clinical decision errors can be identified.

As with the medication kardex review above, it is important to be systematic in your approach so that you don't miss any potential problems for your patient. This step ideally occurs on the ward, although it is also regularly performed in the dispensary.

How to ... clinically check a hospital discharge prescription's accuracy

This can be carried out by a qualified accuracy checking technician or pharmacist.

Stepwise approach to screening (questions to ask yourself)

1. Check the age of the patient.
   a. If the prescription is for a child:
      i. Check a recent weight (note date – especially for neonates)
      ii. Check if liquids are needed
2. Check the ward the patient has come from.
   a. E.g. if it is a maternity ward is the patient pregnant or breastfeeding?
3. Check each medication prescribed for appropriateness and safety:
   a. Suitable medication
   b. Suitable dose
   c. Suitable frequency
4. Check that the dosage form is the most appropriate for the patient.
   a. If patients have been diagnosed with a stroke:

     i. Can they swallow oral dosage formulations or do they require an alternative route?

    ii. If another route is required, is it the same salt as the oral dosage form and does it require a dosage adjustment?

5. Check that the dosage form is appropriate for the route it is to be given.
   a. If the drug has been prescribed in an oral dosage form but it is advised to be given intravenously

6. All medicines should be prescribed generically (except where brand prescribing is indicated e.g. theophylline preparations: lithium preparations (not exhaustive)).

7. All short-term medications should have a stop date stated.
   a. For example: antibiotics, electrolyte supplements, short-term prednisolone

8. Have any medications been continued unnecessarily? For example:
   a. Sleeping tablets prescribed in patients who should only receive them in hospital
   b. Nebules prescribed in patients admitted with respiratory problems who do not have nebulisers at home

9. Are there any medications missing based on the patient's diagnosis? For example:
   a. Breakthrough pain relief in a patient receiving a modified release opioid
   b. Laxatives for someone on regular opioids
   c. No anticoagulant in a patient with AF.

10. Is there any therapeutic duplication?
    a. New beta-blocker prescribed and old agent not discontinued
    b. Patient taking a DOAC (Direct Oral Anticoagulant Drug) who is also prescribed enoxaparin

11. Are any of the medications contraindicated based on the patient's diagnosis?
    a. Rate-limiting calcium channel blocker (diltiazem, verapamil) in a patient with heart failure
    b. NSAID (Non Steroidal Anti Inflammatory Drug) in a patient with a diagnosis of GI bleed

12. Are any of the prescribed medications considered 'high risk' or a 'trigger' drug?
    a. Do they require more thorough consideration due to a narrow therapeutic index for example digoxin, warfarin?
    b. Do they require caution to their high risk of errors and risk of toxicity, for example methotrexate?

13. Does the medication interact with other medications/disease state/food?

14. Is the patient allergic to any of the medicines prescribed?

15. Check discharge prescription for legalities e.g. ensure prescription is signed (legal requirement).

Example 2

The Hospital		DISCHARGE AND MEDICATION ADVICE LETTER

DR SC GUNN   GP CODE:
GREENFIELDS HC
FAIRVIEW
Magherafelt
BT24 7AD

Mr Carl Hamill
72 The Red Lane
Magherafelt
BT23 9AA

Admission Date:	**22/04/2015**	Phone No:	**02890666666**
Admission Method:	**Via A&E**	DOB:	Age:
Discharge Date:		Sex:	**M**
Discharge Method:	**Discharge to home**	H&C No:	353 684 8960
Ward:	**Ward One**		
Discharging Consultant:	**Dr Marten**		

CURRENT EPISODE DETAILS

Principal Diagnosis:	Fractured elbow
Underlying Conditions & Co-Morbidities:	Bipolar disorder (on lithium), high cholesterol.
Procedures/Dates:	Follow up in 2 weeks at clinic
Relevant Clinical Concerns:	Refer for physiotherapy and prescribe analgesia.

FOLLOW UP PLANS	**COMMENTS**
Outstanding Investigations:	None
Hospital Review Arrangements:	As above – 2 weeks follow up appointment in clinic.
Additional Care Arrangements:	None
Action Required By GP:	Please update medical records accordingly.

Continued

Figure 5.2   Discharge Rx form.

ALLERGY / DRUG SENSITIVITIES	NKDA			TYPE OF REACTION (IF KNOWN)			

MEDICATION ON DISCHARGE

Take home supply needed Y/N	MEDICINE (APPROVED NAME)	ROUTE	DOSE AND FREQUENCY	NOTES / COMMENTS DURATION IF APPROPRIATE, INDICATION IF NEW DRUG, TITRATION ETC.	CHANGES N-New I-Increased D-Decreased	PHARMACY INFORMATION (INCLUDING QUANTITY SUPPLIED)
Y	Lithium	PO	400 mg mane			
Y	Simvastatin	PO	40 mg nocte			
Y	Paracetamol	PO	1Q QDS	Doses must be a minimum of 4 hours apart.	N	

MEDICATION STOPPED	REASON FOR STOPPING

ADDITIONAL MEDICATION INFORMATION

PHARMACY ONLY	INITIAL AND DATE
Clinical Check in Dispensary	
Clinical Check at Ward Level by CP	
Labelled / Dispensed	
Checked	
Medication Card Required	No

Comments
All medications reconciled on discharge by a clinical pharmacist Y or N

Prescribed by C Smith PIP 3357
Pharmacist Independent Prescriber

(Signature) ...... C Smith ......
GMC Number

Date:
Grade: PIP
Bleep No: 239

Figure 5.2—cont'd

Issues identified

1. No DOB on the prescription – this would have to be highlighted to a prescriber or to confirm from patient notes if on the ward.
2. The Prescription has not been dated – this must be added by the prescriber.
3. Lithium has been prescribed generically and as per BNF, the bioavailability of lithium preparations vary widely and brand prescribing is required – you will need to identify this to the prescriber and ask for this to amended prior to dispensing.
4. What did the patient receive during their admission? Did they receive the appropriate brand? Advise that a lithium level should be requested to confirm the level is within the normal range, the range could be provided to the prescriber also e.g. 0.4–1 mmol/L (this may vary depending on the laboratory used).
5. Review the patient's analgesia requirements prior to discharge and advise appropriate medication if required.
6. Consider completing an incident report form or equivalent for the inappropriate prescribing of lithium.

Example 3

The Hospital	DISCHARGE AND MEDICATION ADVICE LETTER

DR NAME + ADDRESS
      GP CODE: 1234

Dr. Murphy
The Surgery

		Patient Name:	EK
		Patient Address:	13 Clonard Walk

Admission Date:	**30/06/2016**	Phone No:	**02890666666**
Admission Method:	**Via A&E**	DOB: 13/07/52	Age:
Discharge Date:		Sex:	**M /(F)**(delete as applicable)
Discharge Method:	**Discharge to home**	H&C No:	353 684 8960
Ward:	**Ward One**		
Discharging Consultant:	**Dr. Riddell**		

CURRENT EPISODE DETAILS

Principal Diagnosis:	Cellulitis
Underlying Conditions & Co-Morbidities:	Acute kidney injury
Procedures/Dates:	
Relevant clinical concerns:	Pain control

FOLLOW UP PLANS	COMMENTS
Outstanding Investigations:	
Hospital Review Arrangements:	
Additional Care Arrangements:	
Action Required By GP:	

Figure 5.3 Discharge prescription for Mrs EK.

| ALLERGY/DRUG SENSITIVITIES | NKDA | | | TYPE OF REACTION (IF KNOWN) | | |

MEDICATION ON DISCHARGE

Take home supply needed Y/N	MEDICINE (APPROVED NAME)	ROUTE	DOSE AND FREQUENCY	NOTES / COMMENTS DURATION IF APPROPRIATE, INDICATION IF NEW DRUG, TITRATION ETC.	CHANGES N-New I-Increased D-Decreased	PHARMACY INFORMATION (INCLUDING QUANTITY SUPPLIED)
Y	Sodium fusidate	0	500mg TID		N	
Y	Flucloxacillin	0	500mg QID		N	
N	Pregabalin	0	75mg BD			
Y	Sando K	0	one BD		N	
N	Esomeprazole	0	40mg	PRN		
Y	Paracetamol	0	1g 4–6 hourly	PRN	N	
Y	Cyclizine	0	50mg 8 hrly	PRN	N	
Y	Diclofenac	0	50mg TID	PRN		

MEDICATION STOPPED	REASON FOR STOPPING

ADDITIONAL MEDICATION INFORMATION

PHARMACY ONLY	INITIAL AND DATE
Clinical Check in dispensary	
Clinical Check at ward level by CP	
Labelled/Dispensed	
Checked	
Medication Card Required	

Comments
All medications reconciled on discharge by a clinical pharmacist Y or (N)

Prescribed by	Date:	2/7/2016
	Grade:	F1
	Bleep No:	2364

(Signature) *Peter Bran*
GMC Number

Figure 5.3—cont'd

Issues identified

1. No duration specified for antibiotics (sodium fusidate and flucloxacillin).
2. No duration specified for Sando K (potassium supplementation, would require K monitoring regularly so usually number of days specified, when querying this with a prescriber, you should know what the target K is and how much potassium is in the Sando K tablets).
3. Esomeprazole prescribed when required. This is usually taken regularly once a day – need to discuss with prescriber to address this issue.
4. Patient was admitted with acute kidney injury (AKI), therefore diclofenac should be held as it can cause AKI, but you may wish to consider an alternative analgesic, so find out what it was prescribed for and make a suitable recommendation.
5. What is the current level of renal function? Do any medicines require dose adjustment? e.g. check pregabalin dose with respect to renal function.
6. Clinically significant interaction between statin and sodium fusidate where risk of rhabdomyolysis is increased – patient should be advised to temporarily discontinue statin whilst taking sodium fusidate and for 7 days after cessation of this antibiotic. They should be advised to report any unexplained muscle pain to GP.

As part of your proprietary dispensing teaching you may have been using a checking framework or developed your own, based on the information provided above. You should employ this framework when completing an accuracy and clinical check on a dispensed prescription.

As part of the 'clinical check' you will look out for drug interactions in your patient's prescription. The following 'how to' guide helps you to identify and offer resolution to drug interactions should you identify them in your clinical screen of a medication kardex or discharge prescription.

How to ... manage a drug interaction

Medications can interact with other drugs, food, disease states or laboratory tests. It is important to know how to identify drug interactions and how to manage these in practice.

Identification and management of drug interactions

On qualification, as you become more experienced, you will come to know many drug interactions 'off the top of your head'. However, even experienced clinical pharmacists should always screen a prescription or medication kardex and check whether there are any drug interactions, using appropriate resources, then offer advice on management.

Sources of information

Appendix 1 of BNF
Appendix 1 in the BNF details drug-drug and some drug–food (cranberry juice, grapefruit juice) interactions. It does not provide any detail on the significance of the interaction or the likelihood of its occurrence.

Stockley's Drug Interactions
Stockley's Drug Interactions offers further information including case reports documenting the interaction, the mechanism of the interaction as well as management advice.
Management advice can include:

- To temporarily discontinue one drug when another is co-prescribed, for example simvastatin on initiation of clarithromycin or fusidic acid
- To alter the dose of one drug on initiation of another, for example reducing theophylline dose by 50% e.g. if the original dose is 400 mg – the new recommended dose would be 200 mg, when ciprofloxacin is prescribed
- To separate the administration times of both medicines when co-prescribed, for example ciprofloxacin and iron
- In some cases, increasing monitoring is the only action required e.g. monitoring the international normalized ratio (INR) and adjusting the warfarin dose on initiation of metronidazole, and rechecking INR and readjusting warfarin dose on metronidazole cessation
- If no clinically significant interaction occurs, no action may be required.

Summary of product characteristics (SPCs)
Information is also available in the SPCs for the medicine (available at www.medicines.org.uk).

If asked to screen a prescription or kardex in your OSCE, *always* check for the possibility of drug interactions, briefly state what each interaction is and the clinical effect and offer management advice. You are not expected to describe great detail about whether the interaction is pharmacokinetic/pharmacodynamic, enzymes involved etc. however in the future, another healthcare professional may expect you to explain this at that level of detail.

Communication
Written
When you have identified a PCI from a medication kardex or a discharge prescription, or a medicines reconciliation form – you may need to enter this information into the patient's multi-professional notes. There are a number of considerations to bear in mind to support the appropriate documentation of PCIs to ensure the patient's care is improved.

How to ... document pharmaceutical care in patient notes

The role of the clinical pharmacist is to ensure the safe and effective use of drugs. As a member of the healthcare team the clinical pharmacist must document pharmaceutical care provided.

Documentation in patient notes should be used for the communication of important information in instances where it has not been possible to adequately amend the prescription through verbal contact with the prescriber or where clarity on the verbal discussion is required for other members of the team.

Writing in the patient notes should not replace verbal discussions with the healthcare team; however verbal communication with individuals does not allow dissemination of the information to other care providers who were not involved in the conversation. Such interventions should be documented in the patient notes as soon as possible.

As well as documenting patient care and progress, patient notes are also used for the following:
- Legal proceedings
- Education
- Research
- Quality Assurance Evaluation.

What should be documented in patient notes?

- Summaries of oral consultations with other team members regarding the patient's drug therapy
- Responses to specific queries
- Information relating to patient's care obtained as a result of medicines information queries
- Recommendations for adjustments to drug dose, dose frequency, dosage form or route of administration not achievable by endorsement of the prescription or contact with the prescriber; actual or potential drug-related problems that warrant surveillance
- A full report on near-miss medication incidents that have 'potential severity' assigned as moderate, major or catastrophic.
- Drug therapy monitoring findings including:
  - The therapeutic appropriateness of the patient's drug regimen
  - Therapeutic duplication
  - Actual or potential interactions
  - Actual or potential drug toxicity and adverse effects

- • Clinical pharmacokinetic lab data relevant to the drug regimen
- • Physical and clinical symptoms relevant to drug therapy
- Patient education and counselling provided

Format of entries in patient notes

- Documentation must be clear, legible and made in black ink.
- Acts must be documented correctly, concisely and objectively.
- Patient's notes are a legal document. Pharmacists must be aware of all of the relevant information before making an entry in the patient notes and are accountable for the accuracy of the entry.
- Pharmacists must not use judgmental language or words that may imply blame or substandard care.
- Recommendations should be documented more subtly than factual findings e.g. using phrases like *'may want to consider'* or *'please consider review'*
- If a pharmacist makes a mistake or adds an entry in the wrong patient notes, this should be corrected by striking a line through the entry. If the entry is in the wrong patient notes, add 'Error – entry in wrong patient medical record' and sign and date.

SOAP

The standard format for all case note entries (for any professional group) should follow a SOAP sequence:

Subjective relevant patient details
Objective clinical findings
Assessment of situation/problem
Proposed management plan

The standard format for pharmacist entries should follow the framework below.

1. Date and time
2. Title (Clinical Pharmacist)
3. The communication
4. The name and designation of doctor or nurse with whom you have discussed the problem
5. Sign and print your name
6. Your status (Pharmacist)
7. Where you can be reached (Bleep No.).

Example 4

21/12/2016 10.15am Clinical Pharmacist

Trough gentamicin level 20/12/2016 at 1800- 2.5 microgram/L (Target trough<1 microgram/L)

Doses appear to have been administered at the prescribed times and with appropriate dosage interval.

Suggest holding next dose and recheck level after a further 24 hours (1800 on 22/12/2016). If this is <1 microgram/L, dose can be administered.

Discussed with Dr Jameson (bleep 5624).
Thanks, Jane Evans
Pharmacist (Bleep 1764).

Figure 5.4   Example of a pharmacist writing in a patient's medical notes.

Example 5.1. OSCE Station: Medicines Optimisation (3rd year level)

Please read the following information carefully. You have 10 minutes to complete the task.

Background

You are the pharmacist on the Care of the Elderly ward. Mr John McFarland, a 70-year-old man, is admitted with a chest infection.

He is experiencing difficulty swallowing tablets and solid food, but can tolerate a liquidized diet and liquid medication.

The junior doctor (F1) asks you to review all of Mr McFarland's oral medication, which he has difficulty swallowing.

Past medical history

Hypertension

Epilepsy

Osteoarthritis

Medication history

Atenolol tablets 50 mg PO daily.

Epanutin® capsules 300 mg PO daily. Paracetamol tablets 1 g PO QID.

Nil OTC medication.

Nil Known Drug Allergies (NKDA).

Results of investigations

All observations and laboratory parameters normal except: WCC 14.2 (4-11 × 10^9 mg/L).

Inpatient progress

Amoxicillin (PO) is commenced to treat the chest infection.

Task

The F1 doctor on the ward would like you to advise him on how to change Mr McFarland's pre-admission medicines to an **alternative formulation**.

1. Review Mr McFarland's medication kardex, and advise the doctor on alternative formulations for each oral medicine which he will be able to swallow.

2. For each medication, suggest an alternative formulation including strength, dose, frequency and the amount of medicine to be injected with each dose – consider whether any dose adjustments need to be made.

3. Note your recommendations on the answer sheet provided and state any clinical monitoring required.

Please submit your completed medication history to the examiner at the end of the OSCE and do not forget to include your name on the form.

Please do not write on or remove the reference book or other materials provided.

Station props that would be provided

1. Instructions for candidate.

2. Candidate answer sheet.

3. Mark sheet.

4. BNF.

5. Mr McFarland's medication kardex (Fig. 5.5).

OSCE Station: Medicines Optimisation – Answer Sheet (for OSCE 5.1)

Candidate's name:_____

Medicine name	Advice for F1 relating to alternative formulation, strength, dose, frequency, amount of medicine to be injected with each dose and any clinical monitoring required
	Alternative formulation:
	Strength:
	Dose:
	Frequency:
	Amount of medicine to be administered with each dose:
	Clinical monitoring required:

| | | | | WQA7000 Rev. October 2011 |

Medicine Prescription and Administration Record

Rewritten on (date): 1/12/16
Record: 1 of 1

Allergies / Medicine Sensitivities

THIS SECTION MUST BE COMPLETED

Date	Medicine (generic) / Allergen	Type of Reaction	Signature
....	....	....	....

OR

No Known allergies ☑ Please tick
Signature: SPauo Date: 1/12/16

Write in CAPITAL LETTERS or use addressograph

Surname: McFarland
First Names: John
Hospital No: 123456
DOB: 6/11/46   Check identity

Hospital: The Trust   Ward: One
Consultant: Denis
Date of Admission: 1/12/16

Admissions Medicines Reconciliation completed		
Sign: .... Date:		
Discharge prescription ordered by		
Sign: .... Date:		

Weight (Kg)	Date	Height (cm)
78	1/12/16	5'8"

Requirements for Prescribing and Administration

- Nurses must not administer medicines that are improperly or illegibly prescribed.
- Do not prescribe or administer medication if the allergy status is not documented and signed (unless in an emergency).
- Prescribe generically (refer to WHSCT Policy for appropriate use of approved/generic names of medicines).
- Print the full name of the medicine in CAPITALS in black ink. Do not abbreviate medicine names.
- Do not alter existing instructions. Cancel and rewrite any changes in medicine therapy.
- Discontinue any therapy by drawing a diagonal line through the prescription and the remainder of the administration record. Enter the date of discontinuation and signature in the 'Stop' space.
- Do not abbreviate 'micrograms', 'nanograms', 'international units' or units; write in full.
- Prescriber's signatures must be written in full; initials are not acceptable.
- Other prescriptions in use must be referenced on the main prescription record.
- Attach all additional charts to the Medicine Prescription and Administration record.
- The administering nurse(s) must initial each administration.
- All kardexes must be rewritten after 14 days.
- Medicines reconciliation - for each regular or when required medicine, indicate changes made to therapy during stay.
  - On admission, refer to the patient's documented medication history, reconcile medicines on the kardex and circle 'no change', 'increased dose', 'decreased dose' or 'new' medicine accordingly.
  - During patient stay, ensure any subsequent changes are similarly indicated and document the reason in the table below.
  - At discharge, ensure information on medicine changes (including stopped medication) is sent to the GP.

Additional Charts in Use *(please tick)*

Epidural ☐	Intrathecal ☐	Blood Sugar Monitoring ☐	Total Parenteral Nutrition (TPN) ☐	Other (please specify) ☐
Patient Controlled Analgesia ☐	Diabetic Ketoacidosis ☐	Fluid Balance ☐	Oral Anticoagulant ☐	Syringe Driver (please indicate 1 or more) ☐
Insulin ☐	Chemotherapy ☐	Anaesthetic Record ☐	Endoscopy ☐	

Special Instructions / Additional Notes on Medicines / Reason for Medicine Omission *(please sign and date)*

Medicines Reconciliation Record During Patient's Stay

	Medication	Commenced in Hospital (tick if YES)	Stopped in Hospital (tick if YES)	Dose Changed ↑ or ↓	Reason for Medication Change
1					
2					
3					
4					
5					

1   OS17629

Figure 5.5 Medication kardex for OSCE example 5.1 – Mr McFarland.

Regular Non-Injectable Medication
Check allergy status and patient identity

Codes for recording omitted doses
Ⓝ = nil by mouth   Ⓥ = vomiting
Ⓡ = patient refused   Ⓓ = drug not available
Ⓟ = patient not available   Ⓞ = other*
Ⓢ = unable to swallow   ⓄⓇ = Prescribed omission*
*Record reasons in medical/nursing notes.
Take action on omitted doses as appropriate

Write in CAPITAL LETTERS or use addressograph

Surname: McFarland

First Names: John

Consultant: Denis   Ward: One

Hospital No: 123456

D.O.B: 6/11/46   *Check identity*

Year: 2016			Day and Month: →		½	²/₁₂	³/₁₂								
Circle times or enter variable dose/time				▼ ▼											
Medicine Atenolol				06⁰⁰ ✓											
Dose 50mg	**Route** 0	**Start Date** 1/12	**Stop Date**	08⁰⁰											
Special Instructions / Directions			**Signature**	12⁰⁰											
				14⁰⁰											
Medicines Reconciliation (circle)				18⁰⁰											
(No Change) Increased Dose Decreased Dose New															
Signature SParis Print Name S Paris Bleep 5555		Pharmacy		22⁰⁰											
Medicine Phenytoin				06⁰⁰											
Dose 300 mg	**Route** 0	**Start Date** 1/12	**Stop Date**	08⁰⁰											
Special Instructions / Directions * TEVA brand *			**Signature**	12⁰⁰											
				14⁰⁰											
Medicines Reconciliation (circle)				18⁰⁰											
(No Change) Increased Dose Decreased Dose New															
Signature SParis Print Name S Paris Bleep 5555		Pharmacy		22⁰⁰											
Medicine Paracetamol				06⁰⁰											
Dose 1 g	**Route** 0	**Start Date** 1/12	**Stop Date**	08⁰⁰											
Special Instructions / Directions * 4–6 hrly *			**Signature** 12⁰⁰												
				14⁰⁰											
Medicines Reconciliation (circle)				18⁰⁰											
No Change Increased Dose Decreased Dose (New)															
Signature SParis Print Name S Paris Bleep 5555		Pharmacy		22⁰⁰											
Medicine Amoxicillin				06⁰⁰											
Dose 500 mg	**Route** 0	**Start Date** 1/12	**Stop Date**	08⁰⁰											
Special Instructions / Directions			**Signature**	12⁰⁰											
				14⁰⁰											
Medicines Reconciliation (circle)				18⁰⁰											
No Change Increased Dose Decreased Dose (New)															
Signature SParis Print Name S Paris Bleep 5555		Pharmacy		22⁰⁰											
Medicine				06⁰⁰											
Dose	**Route**	**Start Date**	**Stop Date**	08⁰⁰											
Special Instructions / Directions			**Signature**	12⁰⁰											
				14⁰⁰											
Medicines Reconciliation (circle)				18⁰⁰											
No Change Increased Dose Decreased Dose New															
Signature Print Name Bleep		Pharmacy		22⁰⁰											

5

Figure 5.5—cont'd

Medicines Optimisation (written)

Example 5.2. OSCE Station: Medicines Optimisation (3rd or 4th year level)

Please read the following information carefully. You have 10 minutes to complete the task.

Background

You are a pharmacist working on the Medical Admissions Unit (MAU). Mr Jim Graham, a 75-year-old man, is admitted with a suspected urinary tract infection (UTI).

Past medical history

Rheumatoid arthritis (inflammatory arthritis affecting joints)

Hypothyroidism (underfunctioning thyroid gland)

Medication history

Levothyroxine 75 µg mane

Methotrexate 10 mg PO once a week (Sunday mane)

Folic acid 5 mg PO once a week (Tuesday mane)

Nil OTC medication

Nil Known Drug Allergies (NKDA)

Results of Investigations

All laboratory parameters and observations normal except: WCC 14 (4-11 $\times 10^9$ mg/L)

CRP 22 (0-5 mg/L)

Temp 38.8°C (37°C)

MSSU (midstream specimen of urine) positive.

Inpatient progress

The consultant prescribed trimethoprim 200 mg PO bd to treat the UTI.

The hospital antibiotic guidelines suggest 7 days of trimethoprim *or* nitrofurantoin.

Task

1. Review Mr Graham's kardex, considering the information provided above and in the reference sources provided.

2. Identify any **pharmaceutical care issues (excluding venous thromboembolism prophylaxis)** and **actions required to resolve them.**

3. Where care issues are identified, document these on the answer sheet provided.

Please do NOT write on or remove materials provided.

Please submit your answer sheet to the examiner at the end of the OSCE, and do not forget to include your name.

Station props that would be provided

1. Instructions for candidate.

2. Candidate answer sheet.

3. Mark sheet.

4. BNF.

5. 'Oral Methotrexate' guideline.

6. Medication kardex for Mr Graham (Fig. 5.6).

	WQA7000 Rev. October 2011
Medicine Prescription and Administration Record	Rewritten on (date): Record: 1 of 1

Allergies / Medicine Sensitivities

THIS SECTION **MUST** BE COMPLETED

Date	Medicine (generic) / Allergen	Type of Reaction	Signature

OR

No Known allergies ☑ Please tick

Signature: *P.Gray*   Date: 1/12/16

Admissions Medicines Reconciliation completed

Sign: .... Date: ....

Discharge prescription ordered by

Sign: .... Date: ....

Write in CAPITAL LETTERS or use addressograph

Surname: Graham

First Names: Jim

Hospital No: 123456

DOB: 22/5/41   *Check identity*

Hospital: The Trust   Ward: Two

Consultant: Sampson

Date of Admission: 1/12/16

Weight (Kg)	Date	Height (cm)
65	1/12/16	5'3"

Requirements for Prescribing and Administration

- Nurses must not administer medicines that are improperly or illegibly prescribed.
- Do not prescribe or administer medication if the allergy status is not documented and signed (unless in an emergency).
- Prescribe generically (refer to WHSCT Policy for appropriate use of approved/generic names of medicines).
- Print the full name of the medicine in CAPITALS in black ink. Do not abbreviate medicine names.
- Do not alter existing instructions. Cancel and rewrite any changes in medicine therapy.
- Discontinue any therapy by drawing a diagonal line through the prescription and the remainder of the administration record. Enter the date of discontinuation and signature in the 'Stop' space.
- Do not abbreviate 'micrograms', 'nanograms', 'international units' or units; write in full.
- Prescriber's signatures must be written in full; initials are not acceptable.
- Other prescriptions in use must be referenced on the main prescription record.
- Attach all additional charts to the Medicine Prescription and Administration record.
- The administering nurse(s) must initial each administration.
- All kardexes must be rewritten after 14 days.
- Medicines reconciliation - for each regular or when required medicine, indicate changes made to therapy during stay.
  - On admission, refer to the patient's documented medication history, reconcile medicines on the kardex and circle 'no change', 'increased dose', 'decreased dose' or 'new' medicine accordingly.
  - During patient stay, ensure any subsequent changes are similarly indicated and document the reason in the table below.
  - At discharge, ensure information on medicine changes (including stopped medication) is sent to the GP.

Additional Charts in Use *(please tick)*

Epidural ☐	Intrathecal ☐	Blood Sugar Monitoring ☐
Patient Controlled Analgesia ☐	Diabetic Ketoacidosis ☐	Fluid Balance ☐
Insulin ☐	Chemotherapy ☐	Anaesthetic Record ☐

Total Parenteral Nutrition (TPN) ☐	Other (please specify) ☐
Oral Anticoagulant ☐	Syringe Driver (please indicate 1 or more) ☐
Endoscopy ☐	

Special Instructions / Additional Notes on Medicines / Reason for Medicine Omission *(please sign and date)*

Medicines Reconciliation Record During Patient's Stay

	Medication	Commenced in Hospital (tick if YES)	Stopped in Hospital (tick if YES)	Dose Changed ↑ or ↓	Reason for Medication Change
1					
2					
3					
4					
5					

1   OS17629

Figure 5.6 Medication kardex for Mr Graham (for OSCE 5.2).

Continued

Regular Non-Injectable Medication
Check allergy status and patient identity

Codes for recording omitted doses

Ⓝ = nil by mouth   Ⓥ = vomiting
Ⓡ = patient refused   Ⓓ = drug not available
Ⓟ = patient not available   Ⓞ = other*
Ⓢ = unable to swallow   ⒪℗ = Prescribed omission*
*Record reasons in medical/nursing notes.

Take action on omitted doses as appropriate

Write in CAPITAL LETTERS or use addressograph

Surname: Graham
First Names: Jim
Consultant: Sampson   Ward: Two
Hospital No: 123456
D.O.B: 22/5/41   *Check identity*

Year: 2016		Day and Month: →			¹/₂	²/₂	³/₂	⁴/₂						
Circle times or enter variable dose/time														

Medicine Levothyroxine — 06⁰⁰ ✓

Dose 75 micrograms	Route 0	Start Date 1/12	Stop Date	08⁰⁰
Special Instructions / Directions			Signature	12⁰⁰
				14⁰⁰
Medicines Reconciliation (circle)				18⁰⁰
(No Change) Increased Dose / Decreased Dose / New				
Signature Gray Print Name P Gray		Pharmacy	22⁰⁰
Bleep 4132				

Medicine Methotrexate — 06⁰⁰ ✓

Dose 10 mg	Route 0	Start Date 1/12	Stop Date	08⁰⁰
Special Instructions / Directions * Weekly-on Sun *			Signature	12⁰⁰
				14⁰⁰
Medicines Reconciliation (circle)				18⁰⁰
(No Change) Increased Dose / Decreased Dose / New				
Signature Gray Print Name P Gray		Pharmacy	22⁰⁰
Bleep 4132				

Medicine Folic acid — 06⁰⁰ ✓

Dose 5 mg	Route 0	Start Date 1/12	Stop Date	08⁰⁰
Special Instructions / Directions * Weekly-on Tues *			Signature	12⁰⁰
				14⁰⁰
Medicines Reconciliation (circle)				18⁰⁰
(No Change) Increased Dose / Decreased Dose / New				
Signature Gray Print Name P Gray		Pharmacy	22⁰⁰
Bleep 4132				

Medicine Trimethoprim — 06⁰⁰ ✓

Dose 200 mg	Route 0	Start Date 1/12	Stop Date	08⁰⁰
Special Instructions / Directions			Signature	12⁰⁰
				14⁰⁰
Medicines Reconciliation (circle)				(18⁰⁰) ✓
No Change Increased Dose / Decreased Dose / (New)				
Signature Gray Print Name P Gray		Pharmacy	22⁰⁰
Bleep 4132				

Medicine

Dose	Route	Start Date	Stop Date	06⁰⁰
				08⁰⁰
Special Instructions / Directions			Signature	12⁰⁰
				14⁰⁰
Medicines Reconciliation (circle)				18⁰⁰
No Change Increased Dose / Decreased Dose / New				
Signature Print Name		Pharmacy	22⁰⁰
Bleep				

5

Figure 5.6—cont'd

Oral methotrexate guideline (for OSCE 5.2)

Licensed indications:
Rheumatoid arthritis; severe psoriasis unresponsive or intolerant to conventional therapy.

Adult dosage and administration:

> Once weekly dosing – specify day of administration (not Monday).

Dermatology and Rheumatology: dose range is 5 mg to 25 mg once each week.
Dose adjusted by specialist according to response. Doses outside these ranges may be considered with prior agreement of initiating specialist and GP. Lower doses should be used in the frail elderly or if there is significant renal or hepatic impairment.

> Always prescribe methotrexate in multiples of the 2.5 mg tablet strength.
> The 10mg tablets must not be used.

Folic acid:
Dose of 5 mg once each week, taken one to two days after the methotrexate. This may reduce the risk of gastrointestinal and haematological toxicity.

Prescriber responsibilities
- Provide the patient/carer with relevant (written) information on use, side effects and need for monitoring of medication. Advise on need for adequate contraception.
- Provide pre-treatment information as per NPSA and shared care monitoring record booklet and record baseline tests.

> *Baseline tests:*
> - FBC
> - LFT
> - U&E
> - Chest X-ray / Pulmonary function tests may be considered in selected patients.
> - ESR & CRP (Rheumatology & Gastroenterology only)

- Prescribe methotrexate (2.5 mg tablets only) once each week (specify day not Monday; "as required" or "as directed" are unsuitable dosage instructions for oral methotrexate) and folic acid 5 mg.
- Report any adverse drug reactions to initiating specialist and the usual bodies (e.g. MHRA)

> *Ongoing monitoring:*
> - FBC, U&E & LFT:
> - (Rheumatology only) every 2 weeks until 6 weeks after last dose increase and provided it is stable, monthly thereafter.
> - (all other specialties) every week until therapy stabilised, thereafter patients should be monitored every 2–3 months.

Prescriber responsibilities contd.

- Ensure no drug interactions with other medicines
- Check patient is using adequate contraception
- Administer influenza vaccine annually unless otherwise advised
- Check patient has had ONE DOSE of pneumococcal vaccine.
- Ask about oral ulceration/sore throat, unexplained rash or unusual bruising at every Consultation

> *Withhold oral methotrexate and contact specialist if;*
>
> ☐ WCC < 4 × 109/L   ☐ Neutrophils < 2 × 109/L
> ☐ Platelets < 150 × 109/L
> ☐ AST / ALT > 2 times the upper limit of normal (minor elevations of AST/ALT are common)
> ☐ Creatinine > 2 times the baseline result   ☐ Oral ulceration / sore throat
> ☐ Unexplained rash / abnormal bruising

Side-effects and cautions

- *Myelosuppression & decreased resistance to infection*: especially respiratory/ urinary tract or shingles/chickenpox. Temporarily withhold methotrexate if patient is systemically unwell with significant infection requiring anti-infective intervention.
- *Hepatotoxicity*: methotrexate may be hepatotoxic, particularly at high dosages.
- *Nausea*: commonly encountered, may resolve with dose reduction and/or addition of anti-emetic medication.
- *Alopecia, stomatitis, diarrhoea*: contact the initiating specialist if severe or persistent.
- *Respiratory function*: infrequently, methotrexate can cause interstitial pneumonitis, pulmonary oedema and fibrosis.
- *Alcohol:* patients are advised that alcohol consumption should be avoided or kept to a minimum, due to the increased potential for liver toxicity.

Contraindications

- Severe renal or hepatic impairment
- Chronic or recurrent infections especially respiratory or urinary tract
- Severe anaemia, leucopenia or thrombocytopenia
- History of alcohol abuse/cirrhosis
- Pregnancy: female patients must be advised not to conceive whilst receiving methotrexate. A reliable form of contraception should be used by men and women whilst on methotrexate and for at least 6 months after discontinuing it.
- Breast Feeding: Women being treated with methotrexate should not breastfeed.
- Vaccines: Live vaccines should be avoided, except on the advice of initiating specialist.

> **!! Do not prescribe concomitant Trimethoprim or Co-trimoxazole !!**
>
> due to risk of pancytopenia

Drug interactions

- Co-prescription of drugs with potential hepatotoxic or nephrotoxic effects is also not advisable
- NSAIDs & Aspirin (<300mg): unlikely to cause any clinically significant adverse effects and treatment can be continued
- Herbal remedies: avoid if possible due to unknown interaction potential.

Medicines Optimisation Answer Sheet (for OSCE 5.2)

Candidate name:		Date:	

Pharmaceutical care issue(s)	Action(s) required to resolve them

Example 5.3. OSCE Station: Opioid Conversion (3rd or 4th year)

Please read the following information carefully. You have 10 minutes to complete the task

Background

You are working on a surgical ward as a pharmacist. Mrs Jemima Spence, a 77-year-old woman, has been admitted for palliative care (dignified and comforting end-of-life care).

Past Medical History

Pancreatic cancer

Social History

Family not coping – hospice care provided.

Medication History

MST Continus® 90 mg bd (modified release morphine)

Oramorph® 30 mg every 4 hours for breakthrough pain (immediate release morphine – patient has not required any doses)

Nil OTC medication

No Known Drug Allergies (NKDA)

Results of investigations

All lab tests and observations normal

Inpatient progress

Patient to be converted from oral medicines to a syringe driver containing diamorphine and metoclopramide.

Task

1. Calculate the **total daily dose of morphine** the patient was taking.

Using the 'Approximate Equivalent Doses of Opioid Analgesics for Adults' guide, establish:

2. The appropriate **dose** of **diamorphine** to include in the syringe driver.

3. The appropriate **dose** and **frequency** of **diamorphine** for breakthrough pain, in case this is required.

4. Document any **changes** that now need to be made to the current drug regime to ensure **patient safety.**

5. List any further **pharmaceutical care issues** and **actions required to resolve them.**

Please do NOT write on or remove materials provided.

Please submit your answer sheet to the examiner at the end of the OSCE, and do not forget to include your name.

Station props that would be provided

Item required

1. Instructions for candidate.

2. Candidate answer sheet.

3. Mark sheet.

4. Laminated copy of 'Approximate Equivalent Doses of Opioid Analgesics for Adults' guide (Fig. 5.7).

5. Calculator.

OSCE Medicines Optimisation – Opioid – Answer sheet (for OSCE 5.3)

Candidate's Name		Date	

Task	Answer
Total daily dose of morphine the patient was taking.	
Dose of **diamorphine** to include in the syringe driver.	
Dose and **frequency** of **diamorphine** for breakthrough pain.	
Changes required to drug regime to **ensure patient safety.**	
Any further **pharmaceutical care issues** and **actions required** to resolve them.	

Approximate Equivalent Doses of Opioid Analgesics for Adults

Use caution when converting opioids in opposite directions as potency ratios may be different.

For conversion between opioids, it is conventional practice to use oral morphine equivalents.

<u>Conversion factors for guidance when converting from one opioid to another.</u>

Oral morphine to **subcutaneous (SC) diamorphine** – Divide by 3
e.g. 30 mg oral morphine = 10 mg SC diamorphine

Oral morphine to **oral oxycodone** – Divide by 2
e.g. 30 mg oral morphine = 15 mg oral oxycodone

Oral morphine to **subcutaneous morphine** – Divide by 2
e.g. 30 mg oral morphine = 15 mg SC morphine

Oral morphine to **oral hydromorphone** – Divide by 7.5
e.g. 30 mg oral morphine = 4 mg oral hydromorphone

Oral oxycodone to **SC oxycodone** – Divide by 2 (Suggested safe practice)
e.g. 10 mg oral oxycodone = 5 mg SC oxycodone

Oral hydromorphone to **SC hydromorphone** – Divide by 2
e.g. 4 mg oral hydromorphone = 2 mg SC hydromorphone

SC diamorphine to **SC oxycodone** – Treat as approximately equivalent up to doses of 60 mg/24 hrs Use caution when converting higher doses (Suggested safe practice)
e.g. 10 mg SC diamorphine = 10 mg SC oxycodone

SC diamorphine to **SC alfentanil** – Divide by 10
e.g. 10 mg SC diamorphine = 1 mg SC alfentanil

SC diamorphine to **SC morphine** – ratio is between 1:1.5 and 1:2 – Multiply by 1.5
e.g. 10 mg SC diamorphine = 15 mg SC morphine

Oral tramadol to **oral morphine** – Divide by 10 (Suggested safe practice)*
e.g. 100 mg oral tramadol = 10 mg oral morphine

Oral codeine / dihydrocodeine to **oral morphine** – Divide by 10
e.g. 240 mg oral codeine / dihydrocodeine = 24 mg oral morphine

ALWAYS REVIEW PATIENT REGULARLY AFTER ANY OPIOID SWITCH AS CONVERSION RATIOS ARE APPROXIMATE AND CONSIDERABLE INTER-PATIENT VARIATION MAY OCCUR.

- Note that dose conversions are approximate only and are given as examples.
- When changing from one opioid to another at high doses or because of toxicity, a dose reduction of 30–50% may be necessary.
- When changing from a sustained release preparation in a patient who has had upper bowel surgery, consider whether there may have been incomplete absorption of the full oral dose.
- Use caution in the elderly and in patients with renal or significant hepatic impairment. Consider reduced doses. In severe renal impairment or dialysis patients, alfentanil may be the preferred opioid. Contact the Palliative Care Team for advice.
- Breakthrough doses for each opioid are calculated as approximately $1/6^{th}$ daily dose (i.e. 4 hourly dose) but lower doses may be used if effective. E.g. for a patient on 60 mg oral morphine over 24 hours, breakthrough dose is 10 mg orally but a lower dose may be effective in some patients.

Figure 5.7 Approximate Equivalent Doses of Opioid Analgesics for Adults.

Example 5.4. OSCE Station: Medicines Optimisation (4th year level)

Please read the following information carefully. You have 10 minutes to complete the task.

Task

Using the Antibiotic Guideline provided:

1. What antibiotic(s) including dose, frequency, duration and route would you recommend for the treatment of moderate cellulitis with known MRSA?

2. Identify any relevant pharmaceutical care issues (excluding venous thromboembolism prophylaxis) and actions required to resolve them.

3. Where care issues are identified, document these on the answer sheet provided.

Please do NOT write on or remove materials provided.

Please submit your answer sheet to the examiner at the end of the OSCE, and do not forget to include your name.

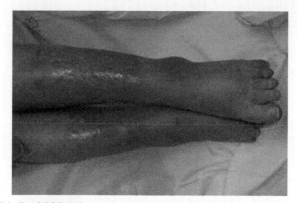

Figure 5.8 Cellulitis (for OSCE 5.4).

Station props that would be provided

1. Instructions for candidate.

2. Candidate answer sheet.

3. Mark sheet.

4. BNF.

5. Antibiotic Guideline for Trust (Fig. 5.9).

INFECTION SYNDROME/INDICATION		PREFERRED REGIMEN Review antibiotic therapy once culture results known	ALTERNATIVE REGIMEN Suitable in serious penicillin allergy	SUGGESTED DURATION	COMMENT
COMMUNITY ACQUIRED PNEUMONIA Pneumonia is typically an acute febrile illness with cough, breathlessness, often productive of sputum and pleurisy in a patient with or without existing chest disease and new shadowing on chest X-ray. Assess severity using **CURB 65** score: new Confusion, Urea >7mmol, Respiratory rate >30/min, **BP** <90 systolic or ≤60 diastolic. **Age ≥65** (Each criterion scores 0 or 1, Therefore, max score = 5).	CURB 65 0-1	Admitted for non-clinical reasons or previously untreated in the community: Amoxicillin 500mg–1g 8 hourly PO	Doxycycline 100mg 12 hourly PO	5–7 days	
	CURB 65 2	Amoxicillin 1g 8 hourly IV/PO. Consider adding Clarithromycin 500mg 12 hourly PO after 48 hours if no improvement	Doxycycline 100mg 12 hourly PO	7 days	
In patients with a CURB-65 score ≥3 with either a history of chronic lung disease or recent treatment with multiple antibiotics, a wider spectrum of cover may be indicated from the outset and the prescriber should consult with senior clinician or microbiologist	CURB 65 3–5 Assess for ICU	Amoxicillin 2g 8 hourly IV **PLUS** Clarithromycin 500mg 12 hourly IV. If there is no response or deterioration within 48 hours change IV Amoxicillin to Co-amoxiclav 1.2g 8 hourly IV	Teicoplanin 10mg/kg 12 hourly IV × 3 doses, then 10mg/kg 24 hourly IV (see TDM section) **PLUS** Clarithromycin 500mg 12 hourly IV	7–10 days	Send blood and sputum cultures. Send pneumococcal and legionella urinary antigen tests.
COMMUNITY ACQUIRED ASPIRATION PNEUMONIA When patients aspirate gastric contents, they develop aspiration pneumonitis for which antimicrobial chemotherapy is **NOT** required. Pneumonitis does not require treatment in first 48 hours unless there is a change in sputum quality to purulent/mucopurulent, fever and new chest x-ray changes which usually occur after 48 hrs.		Amoxicillin 1g 8 hourly IV **PLUS** Metronidazole 500mg 8 hourly IV	Clarithromycin 500mg 12 hourly IV **PLUS** Metronidazole 500mg 8 hourly IV	5–7 days	Only treat if clinical/Chest x-ray evidence of pneumonia.
NON-PNEUMONIC LOWER RESPIRATORY TRACT INFECTION e.g. BRONCHITIS (CHRONIC) OR INFECTIVE EXACERBATION OF COPD No pneumonic changes on chest x-ray. For infective exacerbations of COPD, only prescribe for patients with two of the following: increased shortness of breath, increased sputum volume and/or increased sputum purulence.		**Antibiotic naive:** Amoxicillin 1g 8 hourly PO **Previous/recent antibiotic:** Doxycycline 100mg 12 hourly PO **OR** Clarithromycin 500mg 12 hourly PO/IV This should be guided by previous sputum culture results	Doxycycline 100mg 12 hourly PO **OR** Clarithromycin 500mg 12 hourly PO/IV This should be guided by previous sputum/endotracheal culture results	5–7 days	A cough of less than 2 weeks duration in healthy adults with no co-morbidities or systemic illness does not require antibiotics. Consider antibiotic use in >60 years or if underlying chest disease.
HOSPITAL ACQUIRED PNEUMONIA (Including Hospital Acquired Aspiration Pneumonia) HAP is over diagnosed clinically. HAP diagnosis requires radiological evidence of new pulmonary infiltrates. Alternative diagnoses should be actively excluded.	<4 days post admission	Co-amoxiclav 625mg 8 hourly PO **OR** 1.2g 8 hourly IV depending on the severity of infection	Teicoplanin 10mg/kg 12 hourly IV × 3 doses then 10mg/kg 24 hourly IV (see TDM section) **PLUS** Aztreonam 1g 8 hourly IV **PLUS** Metronidazole 500mg 8 hourly IV This should be guided by previous sputum/endotracheal culture results	5–7 days	Confirmed Pseudomonas or Staph aureus pneumonia may require different therapy with a longer duration. Please seek advice from a microbiologist
	≥4 days post admission	Piperacillin tazobactam 4.5g 8 hourly IV ± Gentamicin 5mg/kg 24 hourly IV (((if severe)) see TDM Section).		5–7 days	
UNCOMPLICATED (LOWER) UTI ASYMPTOMATIC BACTERIURIA: Do not treat unless pregnancy or urology procedures planned.		Trimethoprim 200mg 12 hourly PO **OR** Nitrofurantoin 100mg 6 hourly PO with food		Female: 3 days Male: 7 days	Nitrofurantoin is contraindicated in severe renal impairment.
COMPLICATED (UPPER) UTI		Antibiotic therapy should be guided by relevant urine culture results Gentamicin 5mg/kg 24 hourly IV (see TDM Section) **OR** Piperacillin-tazobactam 4.5g 8 hourly IV depending on the renal function	Antibiotic therapy should be guided by relevant urine culture results. Teicoplanin 10mg/kg 12 hourly IV × 3 doses then 10mg/kg 24 hourly IV (see TDM section) **PLUS EITHER** Gentamicin 5mg/kg 24 hourly IV (see TDM section) **OR** Aztreonam 1g 8 hourly IV	7–10 days Pyelonephritis: 14 days	Review gentamicin requirement on day 3–4 for suitable oral alternative based on the clinical condition and antibiograms.
CATHETER ASSOCIATED UTI Patients with urinary catheter invariably develop bacteriuria after a few days. However, treatment with an antibiotic is required **only** if there are signs and symptoms of systemic infection.		Antibiotic therapy should be guided by relevant urine culture results Gentamicin 5mg/kg 24 hourly IV (see TDM section)		7–10 days Duration depends on severity of infection	Review gentamicin requirement at day 3. Re-assess need for catheter. If it is required consider changing under antibiotic cover.

Figure 5.9 Antibiotic guidelines (for OSCE 5.4).

Condition	First-line treatment	Alternative	Duration	Comments
NEUTROPENIC SEPSIS Neutrophil count of <1 × 10^9/L + Temp >38°C.	Piperacillin/tazobactam 4.5g 6 hourly IV ± Gentamicin 5mg/kg 24 hourly IV (see TDM section) **In severe sepsis add** Teicoplanin 10mg/kg 12 hourly IV × 3 doses, then 10mg/kg 24 hourly IV (see TDM section)	Ciprofloxacin 600mg 12 hourly IV **PLUS** Gentamicin 5mg/kg 24 hourly IV (see TDM section) **PLUS** Teicoplanin 10mg/kg 12 hourly IV × 3 doses, then 10mg/kg 24 hourly IV (see TDM section)	7–14 days Depending on severity	If no improvement after 24 hours discuss with relevant oncologist/haematologist.
SEPSIS OF UNKNOWN ORIGIN SEPSIS Criteria: Clinical impression of infection + 2 of: Temp >38°C or <36°C, pulse > 90bpm, resp rate >20/min, WCC >12 or <4 × 10^9/L. SEVERE SEPSIS: Sepsis + organ dysfunction or hypoperfusion or hypotension.	Piperacillin-tazobactam 4.5g 8 hourly IV ± Gentamicin 5mg/kg 24 hourly IV (see TDM section) Known MRSA Carrier: Add Teicoplanin 10mg/kg 12 hourly IV × 3 doses, then 10mg/kg 24 hourly IV (see TDM section)	Teicoplanin 10mg/kg 12 hourly IV × 3 doses then 10mg/kg 24 hourly IV **PLUS** Gentamicin 5mg/kg 24 hourly IV (see TDM section) **PLUS** Metronidazole 500mg 8 hourly IV	7–14 days Depending on severity	
INTRA-ABDOMINAL SEPSIS (Including biliary tract infections)	**Moderate:** Community acquired non-severe: Co-amoxiclav 1.2g 8 hourly IV **Severe:** Hospital acquired/Complicated: Piperacillin-tazobactam 4.5g 8 hourly IV ± Gentamicin 5mg/kg 24 hourly IV (see TDM section)	Teicoplanin 10mg/kg 12 hourly IV × 3 doses then 10mg/kg 24 hourly IV (see TDM section) **PLUS** Metronidazole 500mg 8 hourly IV **PLUS EITHER** Gentamicin 5mg/kg 24 hourly IV (see TDM section) **OR** Aztreonam 1g 8 hourly IV	5–10 days Depends on source & severity	
CELLULITIS/SOFT TISSUE INFECTION: NO MRSA **Mild:** no signs of systemic toxicity, have no uncontrolled co-morbidity. **Moderate:** either systemically well but with a co-morbidity e.g. peripheral vascular disease, chronic venous insufficiency or morbid obesity which may complicate or delay resolution of their infection OR may have significant systemic upset such as acute confusion, tachycardia, tachypnoea, hypotension, or may have unstable co-morbidities that may interfere with a response to therapy or have a limb, threatening infection due to vascular compromise. Severe sepsis syndrome or severe life threatening infection e.g. necrotising fasciitis (see comments section)	**Mild:** Flucloxacillin 500mg–1g 6 hourly PO. Add Amoxicillin 500mg 8 hourly PO if streptococcal infection is suspected e.g. if cellulitis spreading. **Moderate to Severe:** Flucloxacillin 2g 6 hourly IV **PLUS** Benzylpenicillin 1.2g 4 hourly IV (consider bolus administration where sodium load is a concern) **OR** Flucloxacillin 1g 6 hourly IV **PLUS** Sodium Fusidate 500mg 8 hourly PO Necrotising Fasciitis (see comments section): Seek urgent advice from microbiologist and surgeon.	Doxycycline 100mg 12 hourly PO **Moderate-Severe:** Clindamycin 900mg 6 hourly IV Necrotising Fasciitis (see comments section): Seek urgent advice from microbiologist and surgeon	7–14 days Depending on severity	Bacterial cultures not required for mild/moderate cellulitis. Severe cellulitis/Necrotising Fasciitis: take blood cultures and send wound swab/pus/debrided tissue for culture. Five clinical features of Necrotising Fasciitis: constant pain, bullous lesions, gas in the soft tissues, systemic toxicity and rapid spread along the fascial planes.
CELLULITIS/SOFT TISSUE INFECTIONS: KNOWN MRSA	**Mild:** Doxycycline 100mg 12 hourly PO ± Sodium Fusidate 500mg 8 hourly PO **Moderate:** Teicoplanin 10mg/kg 12 hourly IV × 3 doses then 10mg/kg 24 hourly IV (see TDM section) **PLUS** Sodium Fusidate 500mg 8 hourly PO **Severe:** Urgent advice from surgeon and microbiologist		7–14 days	Prescription must be guided by MRSA antibiogram where known
BACTERIAL MENINGITIS Refer to Empirical Antibiotic Guidelines for Secondary Care within the Policy Library on Staffnet.	Cefotaxime 2g 6 hourly IV **OR** Ceftriaxone 2g 12 hourly IV **If >55 years, immunocompromised or pregnant** add Amoxicillin 2g 4 hourly IV	Chloramphenicol 25mg/kg 6 hourly IV. **If >55 yrs or immunocompromised** add Co-trimoxazole 1.44g 12 hourly IV	Depends on pathogen isolated	Seek consultant advice.
***Clostridium difficile*-Associated Diarrhoea** **Mild/Moderate Disease:** WCC <15 × 10^9/L, CRP <150, Normal Abdominal X-ray. **Severe Disease:** unwell and any one of these, WCC >15 × 10^9/L, CRP >150, Abnormal Abdominal X-ray, Distended Abdomen.	**Mild/Moderate Disease:** Metronidazole 400mg 8 hourly PO. Refer to Empirical Antibiotic Guidelines for Secondary Care within the Policy Library on Staffnet **Severe Disease:** Refer to Empirical Antibiotic Guidelines for Secondary Care within the Policy Library on Staffnet.		10–14 days. Review daily.	Refer to full guidance on the management of Clostridium difficile infection which is available on the ward and in the Empirical antibiotic guidelines for secondary care within the policy library on staffnet.

Figure 5.9—cont'd

OSCE Answer sheet (for OSCE 5.4)

Candidate name:		Date:	

Antibiotic(s) including dose, frequency, duration and route

Pharmaceutical care issue(s)	Action(s) required to resolve them

OSCE station mark sheet (for OSCE 5.1)

Candidate's Name		Date	

Assessment Criteria for Example 5.1:		Mark	
Atenolol			
1. Specify changing formulation to atenolol syrup **(1 mark)** 25 mg/5 ml **(1 mark)**	0	1	2
2. Dose recommended is 50 mg **(1 mark)** once daily **(1 mark)**	0	1	2
3. 10 ml to be administered with each dose	0	1	-
4. Monitor patient e.g. for efficacy *(blood pressure control)* **OR** *bradycardia* **OR** specific side effects such as nausea, vomiting **(1 mark for each point. Maximum 2 marks)**	0	1	2
Epanutin® (Phenytoin)			
5. Specify changing formulation to Epanutin® syrup **(1 mark)** 30 mg/5 mL **(1 mark)**	0	1	2
6. ***Dose recommended is 270 mg daily as an approximate equivalent dose to 300 mg capsule (2 marks)***	0	-	2
7. 45 mL to be administered with each dose **(1 mark)**	0	1	-
8. Monitor patient e.g. for efficacy (seizure frequency) **OR** specific side effects such as nausea, diarrhoea, vomiting **(1 mark for each point. Maximum 2 marks)**	0	1	2
Paracetamol			
9. Specify changing formulation to paracetamol oral suspension or soluble tablets **(1 mark)** 250 mg/5 ml or 500 mg **(1 mark)**	0	1	2
10. Dose recommended is 20 ml of 250 mg/5 ml suspension or 2 of 500 mg tablets four times daily **(1 mark)**	0	1	-
11. Monitor patient e.g. for efficacy (symptom control) **OR** specific side effects such as dyspepsia, vomiting **(1 mark for each point. Maximum 2 marks)**	0	1	2
12. Subtract one mark if candidates suggest 120 mg/5 ml suspension since greater volume for patient to swallow	-1	0	
Amoxicillin			
13. Specify changing formulation to amoxicillin oral suspension **(1 mark)** 250 mg/5 ml **(1 mark)**	0	1	2
14. 10 ml (500 mg) to be administered with every dose **(1 mark)**	0	1	-
Any other valid point (discretionary: only awarded if full marks not obtained elsewhere)			
15. Endorse kardex with details of dose adjustments for phenytoin including volumes to administer etc.	0	1	2
16. Mention the sodium content of paracetamol soluble tablets which need to be considered as the patient has hypertension			
17. Other _____			

Issue(s) relating to patient safety

If candidates propose any course of action which could lead to serious harm or death, they will **fail** the OSCE. Always seek a second opinion. Give detail:

Continued

OSCE station mark sheet (for OSCE 5.1)—cont'd

Total Mark:		/ 22	
Angoff score (borderline competence): 14 Criterion in bold italics is essential (criterion 6 – all aspects)		**Pass**	**Fail**

Assessor's Comments:

Assessor's Signature: _____

OSCE station mark sheet (OSCE 5.2)

Candidate's Name		Date	

Assessment Criteria for Example 5.2:			Mark	

Trimethoprim in UTI

1. Identifies that trimethoprim should not be co-prescribed with methotrexate due to the risk of pancytopenia/haematological toxicity	0	-	2	
2. **Candidate should request that the doctor ceases the trimethoprim on the medication kardex**	0	-	2	
3. Candidate should suggest nitrofurantoin as an alternative antibiotic **(2 marks)** as per hospital guidelines (provided)	0	1	2	
4. Recommends a dose of 50–100 mg **(1 mark)** orally **(1 mark)** four times daily **(1 mark)**	0	1	2	3
5. Candidate should suggest monitoring patient for effect of antibiotic including symptom resolution, reduction in CRP, WCC, temperature etc. **(1 mark for each point. Maximum 2 marks)**	0	1	2	

Methotrexate

6. Recommend holding methotrexate until the infection resolves	0	-	2	
7. Candidate should request that the doctor annotates the kardex to show that the methotrexate has been temporarily held due to the infection	0	-	2	

Any other valid point (discretionary: only awarded if full marks not obtained elsewhere)

8. Completing incident form due to any issue identified above	0	1	2	
9. Counsel the patient on why the trimethoprim was stopped				
10. Counsel the patient on why the methotrexate has been temporarily held				
11. Recommend an annual influenza vaccine				
12. Check how patient manages mediations due to rheumatoid arthritis (RA), if requires non-CRCs				

OSCE station mark sheet (OSCE 5.2)—cont'd

13. Take nitrofurantoin with food		
14. Continue the antibiotic course for 7 days		
15. Recommend routine monitoring of FBC or U&E or LFTs or ESR/CRP when methotrexate recommenced		
16. Other		

Issue(s) relating to patient safety

If candidates propose any course of action which could lead to serious harm or death, they will **fail** the OSCE. Always seek a second opinion. Give detail:

Total Mark	**/ 15 (max)**	
Angoff score (borderline competence): 9 Criteria in bold italics is essential (criterion **2**)	**Pass**	**Fail**

Assessor's Comments:

Assessor's Signature: _____

OSCE station mark sheet (for OSCE 5.3)

Candidate's Name		**Date**	

Assessment Criteria for Example 5.3:	**Mark**		
Total daily dose of morphine the patient was taking			
1. Patient was taking 180 mg of morphine	0	-	4
Dose of diamorphine required in syringe driver			
2. *60 mg of diamorphine should be included in the syringe driver*	0	-	4
Dose of diamorphine for breakthrough pain			
3. 10 mg diamorphine for breakthrough pain	0	-	4
4. Take this every four hours	0	-	2
Discretionary marks (only award if full marks not gained in part 3): 5. Award **2 discretionary marks** if the candidate just states that breakthrough pain dose is 1/6th but does not indicate the numerical value	0	-	2
Changes to drug regime to ensure patient safety			
6. Ensure MST and Oramorph **(1 mark)** are discontinued **(1 mark)**	0	1	2

Continued

OSCE station mark sheet (for OSCE 5.3)—cont'd

Pharmaceutical Care Issues And Action Required to Resolve

	0	1	2	3
Award up to 3 marks for any issue(s) mentioned below: Monitoring parameters e.g. opiate side effects (1 mark) and measures to counteract these (1 mark) (laxatives, antiemetics, dose reduction etc.) Student discusses *any* aspect relating to syringe driver use e.g. measuring volume, checking rate of infusion, ensuring syringe driver chart completed, monitoring infusion site etc. (1 mark)				

Any other valid point up to a maximum of 2 points e.g.

	0	1	2
Adjuvant medicine(s) to manage terminal symptoms e.g. for excess respiratory secretion, restlessness etc. Other_____			

Total Mark:	/21	
Angoff score: 8 Criterion in bold italics is essential (i.e. criterion 2)	Pass	Fail

Assessor's Comments:

Assessor's Signature: _____

OSCE station mark sheet (for OSCE 5.4)

Candidate's Name		Date	

Assessment Criteria for Example 5.4:	Mark		
Teicoplanin for MRSA affected moderate cellulitis			
1. Identifies that intravenous **(1 mark)** teicoplanin **(1 mark)** should be recommended in this case	0	1	2
2. Recommends a loading dose of 10 mg/kg **(1 mark)** equivalent to 520 mg *(500 mg would be used but 520 mg is acceptable)* **(1 mark)**	0	1	2
3. Recommend administration of teicoplanin every 12 hours **(1 mark)** for 3 doses **(1 mark)**	0	1	2
4. Maintenance dose is 10 mg/kg 24 hourly **(1 mark)** or 520 mg for 7–14 days **(1 mark)**	0	1	2
5. *Renally impaired patient – advise normal dose on days 1–4 and then give 500/520 mg every 48 hours thereafter*	0	-	2
6. Teicoplanin levels: trough (pre-dose) **(1 mark)** and expected range 20– 60 mg/L **(1 mark)** take levels earlier due to renal impairment	0	1	2

OSCE station mark sheet (for OSCE 5.4)—cont'd

7. Candidate should suggest monitoring patient for effect of antibiotic including symptom resolution, temperature.	0	-	2

Sodium fusidate

8. Identifies that sodium fusidate is recommended as well as teicoplanin in moderate cellulitis **(2 marks)**	0	-	2
9. Recommends a dose of 500 mg 8 hourly **(1 mark)** orally **(1 mark)**	0	1	2

Any other valid point (discretionary: only awarded if full marks not obtained elsewhere)

10. Monitor temperature/WCC	0	1	2
11. Monitor patient symptoms			
12. Monitor site of infection			
13. Monitor patient re: requirements for pain relief/recommend pain relief			
14. Monitor renal function			
15. Give teicoplanin whilst awaiting trough results			
16. Other_____			

Issue(s) relating to patient safety

If candidate propose any course of action which could lead to serious harm or death, they will **fail** the OSCE. Always seek a second opinion. Give detail:

Total Mark	**/ 18 (max)**	
Angoff score (borderline competence): 9 Criteria in bold italics is essential (criterion 5)	**Pass**	**Fail**

Assessor's Comments:

Assessor's Signature: _____

✔ How to excel in this type of station

Action	Reason	How
Be systematic	If you are e.g. reviewing the medication chart / kardex. Always also look to see if the medication has been given to the patient i.e. has a nurse signed the administration section so you can judge how to act if the patient has actually received the medication or not.	Start at the first page and look at the patient details including allergy status and then move on to the medications prescribed regularly, when required and as once only – checking their doses, frequencies etc.
Self-check any recommendations	It is easy to make an error when reading information from an unfamiliar monograph or guideline, take your time.	If you are e.g. recommending a dose increase or reduction or a change of medication, check your information at least twice to ensure you have documented this clearly for the prescriber.
Self-check any calculations	Dosing errors can lead to non-improvement from under-dose or patient harm if an overdose particularly in extremes of age or weight, particularly if the medication is one with which you are unfamiliar.	If you are familiar with the medication, consider what you think is a reasonable dose for this individual patient; this will help you judge if your calculation appears plausible. For example, if you calculate the rate of a dopamine infusion to be 1,000 ml/hr, is this reasonable? Can this be given to a patient?
Use the resources provided and complete the task as directed.	If a guideline or photocopy from a textbook is provided, it suggests that this is something important for you to consider, but never forget to review the patient information as there may be more than one issue for you to identify and resolve.	If the task asks you to review the dose using the guideline provided, ensure that you do this, however, also review the patient for their co-morbid states, concurrent medications, as you would with a real patient encounter to ensure you have identified all of the risk pertaining to this patient.
Recording your answer in medical note style	This type of OSCE could require you to demonstrate your competency in written communication to other healthcare professionals. It is important to be familiar with the expected format for professional staff recording in patient medical notes as well as ensuring that your suggestions are clear and readily interpretable by the medical staff to whom you are addressing.	You may be asked to record your answer in multiprofessional notes – see Figure 5.4 for support on how to do this.

✗ Common errors in this type of station		
Action	**Remedy**	**Reason**
Recommending medications to which the patient is allergic or unable to receive	You are asked to recommend a suitable antibiotic – check if the patient is allergic to the antibiotic or if there are sensitivities which suggest this agent is suitable or unsuitable for your patient.	If you give an inappropriate or ineffective medication to your patient, they will not improve and you have put them at risk of harm.
Identifying the error e.g. a drug interaction but not recommending a resolution to the risk identified.	If you identify that e.g. the patient has been prescribed simvastatin and amlodipine, ensure that you recommend what you would do for your patient e.g. maximum of 20 mg of simvastatin daily.	It is important to identify what the risk is to the patient, but you also need to recommend how to manage the problem you have identified to ensure the patient does not come to any harm.

Further reading

Royal Pharmaceutical Society. Medicines optimisation: helping patients to make the most of medicines. Good practice guidance for healthcare professionals in England (May 2013). London, RPS, 2013. Retrieved on 18 August 2015 from <www.rpharms.com/promoting-pharmacy-pdfs/helping-patients-make-the-most-of-their-medicines.pdf>.

Consultations skills. Retrieved on 18 August 2015 from <www.consultationskillsforpharmacy.com>.

Hepler, C.D., Strand, L.M., 1990. Opportunities and responsibilities in pharmaceutical care. Am. J. Health Syst. Pharm. 47, 533–543.

Supporting Research and Development in the NHS, 1994. (Culyer Report). A report to the Minister for Health by a Research and Development Task Force. HMSO, London.

Transforming your Care (TYC), 2011: Retrieved on 22 December 2014 from <https://www.health-ni.gov.uk/topics/health-policy/transforming-your-care>.

In order to improve patient care, the modern NHS focusses on a team approach in which healthcare professionals from a variety of backgrounds use their specialist knowledge and skills to significantly improve patient outcomes.

During your career as a pharmacist, you will be expected to interact professionally with a wide range of healthcare professionals, particularly doctors and nurses but including pharmacists working in a range of healthcare settings. There are important characteristics that support effective working relationships including:

- Team members viewing their roles as important to team success
- Team members viewing the roles of others as important to team success
- No barriers to communication
- Autonomy of practice
- Equality of access to resources

It is important to remember that *poor* interprofessional collaboration can have a negative impact on the quality of patient care. You will need to develop and continually evolve your consultation skills, with particular emphasis on negotiation skills, in order to effectively interact with your future colleagues to ensure the best outcome for your patient. You should be given some guidance on communication skills and professionalism during your MPharm degree (and in the earlier chapter on medicines optimisation).

There are some competencies suggested by the Centre for the Advancement of Interprofessional Education (CAIPE) to support effective working relationships between team members:

- Role clarification: Students should understand their role as well as the roles of those in other professions and should use this to appropriately achieve patient care goals.
- Consult with colleagues regarding roles, knowledge, skills and attitudes using appropriate methods including verbal communication and body language.
- Team dynamics
- Students should understand the principles of team work dynamics as well as group interactions to enable effective interprofessional interactions including effective facilitation of discussions, respect for all team members, self and peer reflection, team ethics, confidentiality and professionalism.

Dealing with queries from a prescriber

Verbal

Although a written record is essential to support the decision-making process in the management of a patient, it is vital to discuss the management of the pharmaceutical care issues with the multi-professional team. The key to interacting with the 'patient' or 'healthcare professional' at the verbal OSCE station is to relate to them exactly as you would with real-life patients or healthcare professionals. In an OSCE, you are expected to communicate in an empathetic manner and answer any questions that they might have.

How to ... interact with a doctor

When screening a prescription or medication kardex and identifying issues requiring resolution e.g. prescription/aspects of kardex not signed; patient prescribed medicine to which allergic; clinically significant drug-drug/disease/food interaction; incorrect dose/frequency; therapeutic duplication; inappropriate dose with respect to co-morbid states e.g. renal function etc. you need to contact the prescriber by telephone or face to face.

A few tips are detailed below.

Telephone conversation

- Introduce yourself (give your name and position).
- Confirm prescriber's identity (as indicated in your task sheet).
- Clearly explain reason for phone call, describing the patient to which query relates using the patient's name and another unique identifier.
- Explain nature of query and suggestion(s) for resolution.
- Remember that if you are not a qualified independent prescriber you are **not legally permitted to make any changes** to the medicine kardex/prescription.
  - You should request that the prescriber makes any of these suggested changes.
- Anticipate further questions; for example if you state that NSAIDs are inappropriate for a patient with cardiovascular disease, the prescriber may ask you to explain why and/or suggest an alternative form of analgesia.
  - If you have not considered these questions, you will look unprepared and unprofessional.
- Aim to address all queries with a single telephone call.
  - If you call the prescriber back, you will appear disorganised and unprofessional.
- On finishing the conversation, thank the prescriber for his/her time.

Some additional tips

- Throughout the conversation, conduct yourself in an appropriately assertive manner, that is, aim to get your point across without being too meek, for example "sorry to bother you" or aggressive, for example "I need to speak to you about mistakes you made". Neither of these approaches is suitable.
- Speak clearly and audibly.
- If a prescriber is rude to you in practice, do not respond in a similar vein, remain calm. If serious, this can be subsequently addressed with the prescriber and the prescriber's line manager.

Face to face conversation

- Introduce yourself (give your name and position).
  - In practice – if prescriber knows you, you do not always need to do this.
- Confirm prescriber's identity – in practice, if you know the prescriber, you will not always need to do this.
- Clearly explain the reason for conversation i.e. patient to which query relates using the patient's name and another unique identifier.
- Explain the nature of query and suggestion for resolution.
- Remember that if you are not a qualified independent prescriber you are **not legally permitted to make any changes** to the medicine kardex/prescription. You should request that the prescriber makes these changes.

- Anticipate further questions e.g. if you state that NSAIDS are inappropriate for a patient with cardiovascular disease, the prescriber may ask you to explain why and/or suggest an alternative form of analgesia. If you have not considered these questions, you will look unprofessional.
- Address all queries in a single setting – if you keep running back to the prescriber, you will appear disorganised and unprofessional.
- On finishing the conversation, thank the prescriber for his/her time.
- Conduct the conversation in an appropriately assertive manner i.e. get your point across without being too meek e.g. "sorry to bother you" or aggressive e.g. "I need to speak to you about mistakes you made". Neither of these approaches are suitable.
- Speak clearly and audibly.
- If a prescriber is rude to you in practice, do not be rude back – remain calm. If serious, this can be subsequently addressed with the prescriber and the prescriber's line manager.

These are the types of competencies which may be included in Doctor interaction OSCEs, they will vary depending on the topic and task required in the OSCE time period.

Table 6.1

Competency		Third year	Fourth year
10.2.1.e	Collaborate with patients, the public and other healthcare professionals to improve patient outcomes	*shows how*	*shows how*
10.2.1 (h)	Provide evidence-based medicines information	*shows how*	*shows how*
10.2.2 (c)	Instruct patients in the safe and effective use of their medicines and devices	*shows how*	*shows how*
10.2.2.d	Analyse prescriptions for validity and clarity	*shows how*	*shows how*
10.2.2 (f)	provide, monitor and modify prescribed treatment to maximise health outcomes	*shows how*	*shows how*
10.2.2.g	Communicate with patients about their prescribed treatment	*shows how*	*shows how*
10.2.2 (h)	optimise treatment for individual patient needs in collaboration with the prescriber	*shows how*	*shows how*
10.2.2.j	Supply medicines safely and efficiently, consistently within legal requirements and best professional practice	*shows how*	*shows how*
10.2.3 (c)	use pharmaceutical calculations to verify the safety of doses and administration rates	*shows how*	*shows how*
10.2.4 (h)	Provide accurate written or oral information appropriate to the needs of patients, the public or other healthcare professionals	*shows how*	*shows how*
10.2.5 (a)	Demonstrate the characteristics of a prospective professional pharmacist as set out in relevant codes of conduct and behaviour	*Does*	*Does*

👥 Buddy activity

Example 6.1.   OSCE Station: Doctor Interaction (4th year)

Please read the following information carefully. You have 10 minutes to complete the task.

Background

You are a pharmacist working on the rheumatology ward. Mr Edward Baird, a 36-year-old man is admitted following a severe flare-up of his rheumatoid arthritis.

Past medical history

Rheumatoid arthritis (inflammatory arthritis involving joints)

Social history

Lives with his wife and 2-month-old daughter.

Medication history (verified by a pharmacist)

Methotrexate 10 mg once weekly on Tuesday

Folic acid 5 mg mane on Thursday

Nil over the counter medication

No known drug allergies.

Results of investigations (from today)

U&Es, FBC, LFTs normal.

CRP 45 (0–6 mg/l).

Inpatient progress

The consultant rheumatologist initiates ibuprofen to provide additional pain relief and reduce inflammation.

Task

1. Review Mr Baird's **medication kardex** considering the information provided above.

2. Identify any **pharmaceutical care issues** and the actions required to resolve them **(excluding venous thromboembolism prophylaxis).**

3. Talk **in person** to **Dr O'Neill** to discuss the care issues which need to be addressed.

You are not qualified as a pharmacist prescriber.

There are 2 people seated at the OSCE station – the examiner and the doctor.

Introduce yourself to the doctor when you are ready to begin.

Please do NOT write on or remove any of the materials provided.

Please submit your answer sheet to the examiner at the end of the OSCE and do not forget to include your name on the form.

Station props that would be provided

1. Instructions for candidate.
2. Copy of script for doctor actor.
3. Candidate notes sheet.
4. Mark sheet.
5. BNF.
6. **Mr Baird's kardex** (Fig. 6.1)

Medicine Prescription and Administration Record	WQA7000 Rev. October 2011 Rewritten on (date): ____ Record: 1 of 1

Allergies / Medicine Sensitivities

THIS SECTION **MUST** BE COMPLETED

Date	Medicine (generic) / Allergen	Type of Reaction	Signature
....	....	....	....
....	....	....	....
....	....	....	....
....	....	....	....

OR

No Known allergies ☑ Please tick

Signature: *H Partridge* .... Date: 1/12/16

Write in CAPITAL LETTERS or use addressograph

Surname: ___Baird___

First Names: ___Edward___

Hospital No: ___123456___

DOB: ___2/3/80___ *Check Identity*

Hospital: ___The Trust___ Ward: ___Three___

Consultant: ___McKinley___

Date of Admission: ___1/12/16___

Admissions Medicines Reconciliation completed

Sign: .... Date: ....

Discharge prescription ordered by

Sign: .... Date: ....

Weight (Kg)	Date	Height (cm)
72	1/12/16	5'11"

Requirements for Prescribing and Administration

- Nurses must not administer medicines that are improperly or illegibly prescribed.
- Do not prescribe or administer medication if the allergy status is not documented and signed (unless in an emergency).
- Prescribe generically (refer to WHSCT Policy for appropriate use of approved/generic names of medicines).
- Print the full name of the medicine in CAPITALS in black ink. Do not abbreviate medicine names.
- Do not alter existing instructions. Cancel and rewrite any changes in medicine therapy.
- Discontinue any therapy by drawing a diagonal line through the prescription and the remainder of the administration record. Enter the date of discontinuation and signature in the 'Stop' space.
- Do not abbreviate 'micrograms', 'nanograms', 'international units' or units; write in full.
- Prescriber's signatures must be written in full; initials are not acceptable.
- Other prescriptions in use must be referenced on the main prescription record.
- Attach all additional charts to the Medicine Prescription and Administration record.
- The administering nurse(s) must initial each administration.
- All kardexes must be rewritten after 14 days.
- Medicines reconciliation - for each regular or when required medicine, indicate changes made to therapy during stay.
    - On admission, refer to the patient's documented medication history, reconcile medicines on the kardex and circle 'no change', 'increased dose', 'decreased dose' or 'new' medicine accordingly.
    - During patient stay, ensure any subsequent changes are similarly indicated and document the reason in the table below.
    - At discharge, ensure information on medicine changes (including stopped medication) is sent to the GP.

Additional Charts in Use *(please tick)*

Epidural ☐	Intrathecal ☐	Blood Sugar Monitoring ☐	Total Parenteral Nutrition (TPN) ☐	Other (please specify) ☐
Patient Controlled Analgesia ☐	Diabetic Ketoacidosis ☐	Fluid Balance ☐	Oral Anticoagulant ☐	Syringe Driver (please indicate 1 or more) ☐
Insulin ☐	Chemotherapy ☐	Anaesthetic Record ☐	Endoscopy ☐	

Special Instructions / Additional Notes on Medicines / Reason for Medicine Omission *(please sign and date)*

Medicines Reconciliation Record During Patient's Stay

	Medication	Commenced in Hospital (tick if YES)	Stopped in Hospital (tick if YES)	Dose Changed ↑ or ↓	Reason for Medication Change
1					
2					
3					
4					
5					

1   OS17629

Figure 6.1 Medication kardex for Edward Baird (for OSCE 6.1).

Regular Non-Injectable Medication
Check allergy status and patient identity

Codes for recording omitted doses

Ⓝ = nil by mouth   Ⓥ = vomiting
Ⓡ = patient refused   Ⓓ = drug not available
Ⓟ = patient not available   Ⓞ = other*
Ⓢ = unable to swallow   ⓄⓇ = Prescribed omission*
*Record reasons in medical/nursing notes.

Take action on omitted doses as appropriate

Write in CAPITAL LETTERS or use addressograph

Surname: Baird
First Names: Edward
Consultant: McKinley   Ward: Three
Hospital No: 123456
D.O.B: 2/3/80   Check identity

Year: 2016			Day and Month: →			½₂	³⁄₁₂	³⁄₁₂						
Circle times or enter variable dose/time				▼	▼									
Medicine Methotrexate					06⁰⁰	PP	SM	PD						
Dose 10 mg	Route 0	Start Date 1/12	Stop Date		08⁰⁰									
Special Instructions / Directions			Signature		12⁰⁰									
					14⁰⁰									
Medicines Reconciliation (circle)					18⁰⁰									
No Change Increased Dose Decreased Dose New														
Signature M.Pak Print Name M Partridge			Pharmacy SP		22⁰⁰									
Medicine Folic acid					06⁰⁰	PP	SM	PD						
Dose 5 mg	Route 0	Start Date 1/12	Stop Date		08⁰⁰									
Special Instructions / Directions			Signature		12⁰⁰									
					14⁰⁰									
Medicines Reconciliation (circle)					18⁰⁰									
No Change Increased Dose Decreased Dose New														
Signature M.Pak Print Name M Partridge			Pharmacy SP		22⁰⁰									
Medicine Ibuprofen					06⁰⁰	PP	SM	RM						
Dose 400 mg	Route 0	Start Date 1/12	Stop Date		08⁰⁰									
Special Instructions / Directions			Signature		12⁰⁰									
					14⁰⁰	SM	—							
Medicines Reconciliation (circle)					18⁰⁰									
No Change Increased Dose Decreased Dose New														
Signature M.Pak Print Name M Partridge			Pharmacy		22⁰⁰	PD	—							
Medicine					06⁰⁰									
Dose	Route	Start Date	Stop Date		08⁰⁰									
Special Instructions / Directions			Signature		12⁰⁰									
					14⁰⁰									
Medicines Reconciliation (circle)					18⁰⁰									
No Change Increased Dose Decreased Dose New														
Signature Print Name Bleep			Pharmacy		22⁰⁰									
Medicine					06⁰⁰									
Dose	Route	Start Date	Stop Date		08⁰⁰									
Special Instructions / Directions			Signature		12⁰⁰									
					14⁰⁰									
Medicines Reconciliation (circle)					18⁰⁰									
No Change Increased Dose Decreased Dose New														
Signature Print Name Bleep			Pharmacy		22⁰⁰									

5

Figure 6.1—cont'd

OSCE (Doctor Interaction) – Dr O'Neill's script (for OSCE 6.1)

If the candidate asks you if you are Dr O'Neill confirm that you are.

The candidates should identify themselves also, if they don't, ask who they are.

If the candidate highlights that methotrexate is prescribed every day and should be once a week, say...

'Oh dear! I cannot believe I prescribed it daily, must have been distracted – you are quite right! I will complete an incident form.' (*The candidate needs to ask you to amend dose frequency on prescription.*)

If the candidate highlights that ibuprofen prescribed interacts with methotrexate, say...

'I know that, but Edward really needs the NSAID for additional anti-inflammatory effect, his renal function, bloods and LFTs are normal and we were just going to monitor his methotrexate closely whilst on the ibuprofen – are there any NSAIDs which do not interact with methotrexate to the same extent as ibuprofen that may be "safer" for me to prescribe instead?'

If the candidate does not know, say...

'Oh right – thought you pharmacists were the medicines experts.'

If the candidate suggests a NSAID which interacts less (e.g. celecoxib, meloxicam, piroxicam (piroxicam restrictions on use but can be used by rheumatologists), say...

'OK – useful to know, I will change him over to XXXXXX.' (Select an NSAID they suggested.)

If the candidate suggests paracetamol/weak opioid, say...

'No, I will not go for either of these – there's not much anti-inflammatory effect to be gained!'

If the candidate highlights that folic acid is prescribed every day, say...

'What is the problem with that? It will reduce the side effects of methotrexate.' (*candidate needs to tell you it should not be taken on the same day as methotrexate and ask you to change frequency – if the candidate does this, agree.*)

If the candidate highlights anything else that you do not consider to be important/relevant, say...

'That's not important, leave it as it is.'

OSCE (Dr Interaction) – Answer sheet (for OSCE 6.1)

Candidate name:		Date:	

Use the space below to make any notes on pharmaceutical care issues you wish to address before speaking with the doctor.
This notes page is submitted but it is **not** assessed.
You are **only assessed** on what you **say to the doctor, as well as your communication style.**

Pharmaceutical Care Issue(s)	Action(s) Required to Resolve this

👥 Buddy activity

Example 6.2.   OSCE Station: Doctor Interaction (4th year)

Please read the following information carefully. You have 10 minutes to complete the task.

Background:

You are the pharmacist working on the admissions ward.

Ms Christine Toba, a 32-year-old woman was admitted with recurring headaches and dizziness.

She is diagnosed with hypertension.

Past medical/surgical history:

18 weeks pregnant

Severe depression (taking citalopram for 8 years including through previous pregnancy; benefit deemed to outweigh risk)

Occasional pregnancy-related constipation

Eczema

Dry eyes

Medication history (which you verified using 2 sources – the patient's own medicines and the patient):

Citalopram 20 mg tablets, one tablet daily

Lactulose solution, 15 ml twice daily

Diprobase cream, apply to hands twice daily

Sodium chloride 0.9% eye drops, one drop in each eye up to four times daily when required for dry eyes

No known drug allergies

All laboratory results and observations are normal except:

BP 158/102 mmHg (<135/85 mmHg)

Inpatient progress:

Christine Toba has been reviewed on the ward round. An analgesic has been prescribed to help alleviate the pain of her headaches, and an antihypertensive for her hypertension.

Task

1. Review Ms Toba's **medication kardex** considering the information provided above.

2. Identify any **pharmaceutical care issues** and the actions required to resolve them (excluding venous thromboembolism prophylaxis).

3. Talk **in person** to **Dr Sampson** to discuss the care issues which need to be addressed.

You are not qualified as a pharmacist prescriber.

There are 2 people seated at the OSCE station – the examiner and the doctor.

Introduce yourself to the doctor when you are ready to begin.

Please submit your answer sheet to the examiner at the end of the OSCE and do not forget to include your name.

DO NOT write on or remove any materials provided.

Station props that would be provided

Item required:

1. Instructions for candidate.

2. Copy of instructions for examiner (observer).

3. Copy of instructions for doctor actor.

4. Script for doctor actor.

5. Candidate notes sheet.

6. Mark sheet.

7. BNF.

8. Ms Christine Toba's kardex (Fig. 6.2)

WQA7000 Rev. October 2011

Medicine Prescription and Administration Record

Rewritten on (date):
Record: 1 of 1

Allergies / Medicine Sensitivities

THIS SECTION **MUST** BE COMPLETED

Date	Medicine (generic) / Allergen	Type of Reaction	Signature
....	....	....	....
....	....	....	....
....	....	....	....
....	....	....	....

OR
No Known allergies ☑ Please tick
Signature: *I.Dupe* Date: 1/12/16

Write in CAPITAL LETTERS or use addressograph

Surname: Toba
First Names: Christine
Hospital No: 123456
DOB: 3/8/84   Check identity

Hospital: The Trust   Ward: Four
Consultant: Julius
Date of Admission: 1/12/16

Admissions Medicines Reconciliation completed
Sign: .... Date: ....
Discharge prescription ordered by
Sign: .... Date: ....

Weight (Kg)	Date	Height (cm)
54	1/12/16	5'4"

Requirements for Prescribing and Administration

- Nurses must not administer medicines that are improperly or illegibly prescribed.
- Do not prescribe or administer medication if the allergy status is not documented and signed (unless in an emergency).
- Prescribe generically (refer to WHSCT Policy for appropriate use of approved/generic names of medicines).
- Print the full name of the medicine in CAPITALS in black ink. Do not abbreviate medicine names.
- Do not alter existing instructions. Cancel and rewrite any changes in medicine therapy.
- Discontinue any therapy by drawing a diagonal line through the prescription and the remainder of the administration record. Enter the date of discontinuation and signature in the 'Stop' space.
- Do not abbreviate 'micrograms', 'nanograms', 'international units' or units; write in full.
- Prescriber's signatures must be written in full; initials are not acceptable.
- Other prescriptions in use must be referenced on the main prescription record.
- Attach all additional charts to the Medicine Prescription and Administration record.
- The administering nurse(s) must initial each administration.
- All kardexes must be rewritten after 14 days.
- Medicines reconciliation - for each regular or when required medicine, indicate changes made to therapy during stay.
    - On admission, refer to the patient's documented medication history, reconcile medicines on the kardex and circle 'no change', 'increased dose', 'decreased dose' or 'new' medicine accordingly.
    - During patient stay, ensure any subsequent changes are similarly indicated and document the reason in the table below.
    - At discharge, ensure information on medicine changes (including stopped medication) is sent to the GP.

Additional Charts in Use (please tick)

Epidural ☐	Intrathecal ☐	Blood Sugar Monitoring ☐
Patient Controlled Analgesia ☐	Diabetic Ketoacidosis ☐	Fluid Balance ☐
Insulin ☐	Chemotherapy ☐	Anaesthetic Record ☐

Total Parenteral Nutrition (TPN) ☐
Oral Anticoagulant ☐
Endoscopy ☐

Other (please specify) ☐
Syringe Driver (please indicate 1 or more) ☐

Special Instructions / Additional Notes on Medicines / Reason for Medicine Omission (please sign and date)

Medicines Reconciliation Record During Patient's Stay

	Medication	Commenced in Hospital (tick if YES)	Stopped in Hospital (tick if YES)	Dose Changed ↑ or ↓	Reason for Medication Change
1					
2					
3					
4					
5					

1   OS17629

Figure 6.2   Medication kardex for Christine Toba (for OSCE 6.2)

Regular Non-Injectable Medication
Check allergy status and patient identity

Codes for recording omitted doses

Ⓝ = nil by mouth Ⓥ = vomiting
Ⓡ = patient refused Ⓓ = drug not available
Ⓟ = patient not available Ⓞ = other*
Ⓢ = unable to swallow ⓄⓇ = Prescribed omission*
*Record reasons in medical/nursing notes.

Take action on omitted doses as appropriate

Write in CAPITAL LETTERS or use addressograph

Surname: Toba
First Names: Christine
Consultant: Julius   Ward: Four
Hospital No: 123456
D.O.B: 3/8/84   *Check identity*

Year: 2016			Day and Month: →		1/12											
Circle times or enter variable dose/time																

Medicine: Citalopram

Dose 20 mg	Route 0	Start Date 1/12	Stop Date	06⁰⁰											
				(08⁰⁰) ✓											
Special Instructions / Directions			Signature	12⁰⁰											
				14⁰⁰											

Medicines Reconciliation (circle): (No Change) | Increased Dose | Decreased Dose | New — 18⁰⁰
Signature P.Samf Print Name P.Samson Pharmacy SP Bleep 1235 — 22⁰⁰

Medicine: Lactulose Liquid

Dose 15 mL	Route 0	Start Date 1/12	Stop Date	06⁰⁰											
				(08⁰⁰) ✓											
Special Instructions / Directions			Signature	12⁰⁰											
				14⁰⁰											

Medicines Reconciliation (circle): (No Change) | Increased Dose | Decreased Dose | New — (18⁰⁰) ✓
Signature P.Samf Print Name P.Samson Pharmacy SP Bleep 1235 — 22⁰⁰

Medicine: Candesartan

Dose 8 mg	Route 0	Start Date 1/12	Stop Date	06⁰⁰											
				(08⁰⁰) ✓											
Special Instructions / Directions			Signature	12⁰⁰											
				14⁰⁰											

Medicines Reconciliation (circle): No Change | Increased Dose | Decreased Dose | (New) — 18⁰⁰
Signature P.Samf Print Name P.Samson Pharmacy Bleep 1235 — 22⁰⁰

Medicine:

Dose	Route	Start Date	Stop Date	06⁰⁰											
				08⁰⁰											
Special Instructions / Directions			Signature	12⁰⁰											
				14⁰⁰											

Medicines Reconciliation (circle): No Change | Increased Dose | Decreased Dose | New — 18⁰⁰
Signature Print Name Pharmacy Bleep — 22⁰⁰

Medicine:

Dose	Route	Start Date	Stop Date	06⁰⁰											
				08⁰⁰											
Special Instructions / Directions			Signature	12⁰⁰											
				14⁰⁰											

Medicines Reconciliation (circle): No Change | Increased Dose | Decreased Dose | New — 18⁰⁰
Signature Print Name Pharmacy Bleep — 22⁰⁰

5

Figure 6.2—cont'd

Continued

Abbreviations for frequency

Once daily = od Every morning = om or mane
Twice daily = bd Every night = on or nocte
Three times daily = tds or tid
Four times daily = qds or qid

Write in CAPITAL LETTERS or use addressograph

Surname: Toba

First Names: Christine

Hospital Number: 123456

D.O.B: 3/8/84

As Required Medicines
Check for allergies / drug sensitivities

Medicine			Start Date	Date													
Sodium chloride 0.9%			1/12/16														
Dose One drop	Route TOP	Freq. (max) Q/D	Stop Date	Time													
Signature *P.Surf*			Signature	Dose Route													
Special Instructions / Directions * Each eye * Eye Drops			Pharmacy	Given by													
Medicine Paracetamol tabs			Start Date 1/12/16	Date	½2	½2											
Dose 1 g	Route O	Freq. (max) 4-6 hrly	Stop Date	Time	6 am	12:00											
Signature *P.Surf*			Signature	Dose Route	1 g O	1 g O											
Special Instructions / Directions * Max. 8 daily *			Pharmacy	Given by	PP	SM											
Medicine			Start Date	Date													
Dose	Route	Freq. (max)	Stop Date	Time													
Signature			Signature	Dose Route													
Special Instructions / Directions			Pharmacy	Given by													
Medicine			Start Date	Date													
Dose	Route	Freq. (max)	Stop Date	Time													
Signature			Signature	Dose Route													
Special Instructions / Directions			Pharmacy	Given by													
Medicine			Start Date	Date													
Dose	Route	Freq. (max)	Stop Date	Time													
Signature			Signature	Dose Route													
Special Instructions / Directions			Pharmacy	Given by													
Medicine			Start Date	Date													
Dose	Route	Freq. (max)	Stop Date	Time													
Signature			Signature	Dose Route													
Special Instructions / Directions			Pharmacy	Given by													

Omitted Doses of Medication

Date	Time	Medication, Dose and Route	Reason for omission and action taken	Signature

Figure 6.2—cont'd

Fourth year OSCE – Dr Sampson's script

Background

- You are Dr Sampson, a junior doctor working on the admissions ward when Ms Christine Toba, a 32-year-old woman (DOB: 01-03-83), is admitted with recurring headaches and dizziness and is diagnosed with hypertension.

  – The consultant, Dr Street, suggested starting **candesartan** for hypertension.

- You are monitoring her blood pressure.

- **Issues which the candidate must identify:**

  1. You prescribed the candesartan.

  2. However, you did not take into consideration that **she is pregnant and that candesartan (and other angiotensin-II receptor antagonists)** may cause problems for the foetus and neonate including problems with blood flow, renal function and skull defects.

  3. Although you have prescribed the candesartan, Ms Toba has **not actually received a dose yet**.

  4. You prescribed her pre-admission medicines onto the kardex, but you omitted the Diprobase cream from the kardex.

  5. **Candidate demeanour:**

  -*The candidate should be APPROPRIATELY assertive (not aggressive or too passive), during the conversation;*

  -*They should display appropriate body language, and maintain good eye contact with you.*

Initiation of conversation

If the candidate asks you if you are Dr Sampson, say.....

'Yes, I am'

If the candidate introduces themselves, stating name and position, say....

'Very nice to meet you (*candidate name*)'

If the candidate does not introduce themselves, or state position, say....

'Sorry – who are you?'

If the candidate does not state which patient (Ms Christine Toba; DOB 01-03-83 and/or hospital number) **the query relates to, say......**

'I have seen lots of patients today – which patient does this query concern?'

Issue 1 – Candesartan/ angiotensin-II receptor antagonists are contra-indicated in pregnant women

The candidate should identify that **candesartan has been prescribed but that it cannot be used in pregnant women.**

It can adversely affect fetal and neonatal blood pressure control and renal function. Skull defects and oligohydramnios (deficiency of amniotic fluid) have also been reported.

Candidates are not expected to identify or explain the last adverse effect.

They should **explicitly ask for the candesartan to be stopped or removed from the kardex or** for a safe alternative to be prescribed instead.

The candidate should also suggest completing an incident form.

Continued

Fourth year OSCE – Dr Sampson's script—cont'd

If the candidate highlights that there can be adverse effects for the pregnancy/ fetus/ neonate with candesartan but does not suggest an action (ie. to stop the candesartan or change it to alternative)

'Is that really an issue? Aren't there adverse effects and risks with all medicines?'

If the candidate tells you that this is an issue, say...

'Oh dear! I did not know that....now what do you want me to do then?'

(candidate should tell you that it is an issue, and that the candesartan should be changed to an alternative safe antihypertensive – if they do not know, do not prompt them; if they tell you that it is not an issue, do not look shocked, just accept their advice)

If the candidate specifically says to stop the candesartan on the kardex and/or change it to an alternative, say....

'Thank you, I will alter it on the medication kardex'

Issue 2 – Diprobase not signed on the kardex

If the candidate states that Diprobase cream is omitted from the kardex, (but does not specify the dose frequency OR ask you to prescribe this on the kardex), say.....

'No problem – what's the frequency?'

(Candidate should specify apply to hands twice a day; do not look shocked if they suggest another anything else, just accept their advice)

If the candidate provides you with a frequency, say....

'Thank you – I will add that to the kardex'

If the candidate states that Diprobase cream is omitted from the kardex, (but does not specify the dose frequency but does ask you to prescribe this on the kardex), say.....

'No problem – what's the frequency?'

(Candidate should specify apply to hands twice a day; do not look shocked if they suggest another anything else, just accept their advice)

If the candidate provides you with a frequency, say....

'Thank you – I will add that to the kardex'

If the candidate states that Diprobase cream is omitted from the kardex, (but does state the frequency AND asks you to prescribe this on the kardex), say.....

'No problem – I will add that to the kardex'

(Candidate should specify apply to hands twice a day; do not look shocked if they suggest another anything else, just accept their advice)

Possible further questioning

The candidate may suggest completing an incident form due to the inappropriate prescribing of perindopril – if they do, say...

'No problem'

If the candidate says anything else which is not relevant to the OSCE, or to the provision of pharmaceutical care, say...

'That's not important, leave that as it is'

Closure of conversation

The candidate should thank you for your time.

OSCE Answer sheet (for OSCE 6.2)

Candidate name:		Date:	

Use the space below to make any notes on pharmaceutical care issues you wish to address before speaking with the doctor.

This notes page is submitted but it is **not** assessed.

You are **only assessed** on what you **say to the doctor, as well as your communication style.**

Pharmaceutical Care Issue(s)	Action(s) Required to Resolve this

Ethical dilemmas

Healthcare professionals routinely deal with difficult situations with patients and other healthcare professionals where there is no black or white answer. Clinical decision making is a complex process and ethical dilemmas can be particularly difficult. The bioethics literature has defined ethical dilemmas in terms of 'conflict and choice between values, beliefs and options for action'. Most pharmacy students are introduced to ethical dilemmas in their undergraduate courses at either a uniprofessional or interprofessional level. Your course may have helped you to approach ethical dilemmas using a professional decision-making model or a systematic approach which considers all aspects of the problem and defends the final decision made. One such approach to dilemmas is described in the Medicines, Ethics and Practice Guide under 'professional judgement'. The process of making such a judgement is summarised as follows:

1. Identify the ethical dilemma or professional issue.
2. Gather relevant information.
3. Identify the possible options.
4. Weigh the benefits and risks of each option.
5. Choose an option.
6. Record.

When dealing with an ethical dilemma in practice you should be aware of the Code of Ethics (summarised in Fig. 6.3) and this can be considered in Stage 2 of the above model. As a student you are subject to the Code of Conduct which contains the same seven principles as the General Pharmaceutical Council (GPhC) principles outlined below in Figure 6.3. You should also consider the relevant legislation and professional guidance as well as your own clinical knowledge. Ultimately your primary concern should be for the health and wellbeing of the patient.

This systematic approach can be employed in the next two OSCE stations. The first OSCE station involves an ethical dilemma involving a patient and the second station involves a scenario involving another healthcare professional.

GPhC Standards of Conduct, Ethics and Performance

The Seven Principles as a pharmacy professional. You must:

1. Make patients your first concern.

2. Use your professional judgement in the interests of patients and the public.

3. Show respect for others.

4. Encourage patients and the public to participate in decisions about their care.

5. Develop your professional knowledge and competence.

6. Be honest and trustworthy.

7. Take responsibility for your working practices.

Professional standards of conduct, ethics and performance for pharmacists in Northern Ireland

Principle 1: Always put the patient first

Principle 2: Provide a safe and quality service

Principle 3: Act with professionalism and integrity at all times

Principle 4: Communicate effectively and work properly with colleagues

Principle 5: Maintain and develop your knowledge, skills and competence

Figure 6.3 GPhC and PSNI Codes.

Mapping against GPhC competencies for education

We have mapped our ethical dilemma OSCEs against the GPhC competencies for initial education and training. See Table 6.2 for what is expected depending on the level a student is at in the MPharm course, as can be evaluated via a simulation in OSCE.

Table 6.2			
Competency		**Third year**	**Fourth year**
10.1. (a)	Recognise ethical dilemmas and respond in accordance with relevant codes of conduct	Shows how	Shows how
10.1 (i)	Engage in multidisciplinary team working	Knows how	Knows how
10.2.1 (e)	Collaborate with patients, the public and other healthcare professionals to improve patient outcomes	Knows how	Knows how
10.2.4 (f)	Conclude consultation to ensure a satisfactory outcome	Knows how	Shows how
10.2.4 (h)	Provide accurate written or oral information appropriate to the needs of patients, the public or other healthcare professionals	Knows how	Shows how
10.2.5 (a)	Demonstrate the characteristics of a prospective professional pharmacist as set out in relevant codes of conduct and behaviour	Shows how	Does

Buddy activity

Example 6.3.   OSCE Station – Dealing with an ethical dilemma (4th year)

Please read the following information carefully. You have 10 minutes to complete the task

Background

It is a Saturday morning, and you are the responsible pharmacist in a busy community pharmacy.

You are approached by a concerned and angry-looking customer (Mrs Finbar) who wishes to speak to the pharmacist in private. Mrs Finbar's daughter Sally came in last week to collect a prescription written by Dr Yaqoob. You take the customer to the consultation room.

Task

1. Establish the problem in your initial consultation with Mrs Finbar.

You are **NOT** required to decide if medicines should be stopped, withheld or started and you may pause the consultation to check resources.

2. Discuss the issue appropriately with Mrs Finbar.

3. Document the interaction on the resource provided. You are assessed on what you **say** to **Mrs Finbar**.

You are provided with sources for the discussion, including Mrs Finbar. There are two people seated at the station; the examiner and Mrs Finbar. Introduce yourself to the patient when you are ready to begin.

Please submit your answer sheet to the examiner at the end of the OSCE and do not forget to include your name on the form.

DO NOT write on or remove the patient information leaflet or any other materials provided.

Station props that would be provided

Item required

1. Instructions for candidate.

2. Candidate answer sheet.

3. Mark sheet.

4. BNF.

5. Microgynon® 30 PIL only.

6. RPS Medicines, Ethics and Practice Guide – http://www.rpharms.com/support/mep.asp.

7. Fraser Guidelines for contraceptive prescriptions from NICE: http://cks.nice.org.uk/contraception -assessment#!scenario:3.

OSCE (ethical dilemma) – Script for actor (for OSCE 6.3)

You are Mrs Sheila Finbar, a 50-year-old mother of three. You have discovered a patient information leaflet in your daughter's bedroom whilst cleaning this morning.

Your daughter is 16 years old and you are deeply concerned that she has been prescribed Microgynon® 30 without your knowledge. You have read the leaflet and you know that this is the 'pill'. You suspect your local GP, Dr Yaqoob, has done this.

The GP cannot be contacted as it is a Saturday and you want the pharmacist to check his or her records to see when this was prescribed and by whom. You are extremely angry and upset.

If the candidate asks about the nature of the query/issue, say.....

'I am absolutely horrified! I found this leaflet under my daughter's bed this morning. I know what it is! You need to look at your records and find out for me who prescribed this. It was probably Dr Yaqoob in that surgery down the road'. (*Hand PIL over to candidate.*)

If the candidate asks for the name of your daughter, say...

'Sally, my eldest'

If the candidate asks about the age of your daughter, say...

'She has only just turned 16…but she could have been on these for some time. As her mother I have a right to know who prescribed these for my child.'

If the candidate asks you if your daughter is with you, say...

'No, she is staying with friends this weekend but I am going to get her back home once I find out who has prescribed this.'

If the candidate asks if her daughter is aware of the situation or knows that she is coming to the pharmacy to seek further information, say...

'No, certainly not.'

If the candidate refuses to give you information about the prescriber, say...

'I have rights as a parent to know what has been prescribed for my child'

If the candidate asks if Sally is vulnerable in any way e.g. suffers from a learning difficulty, say...

'No.'

The conversation can be closed with...

If information has been given about the prescriber etc.

'Thanks for this, you have been brilliant.'

If information has not been given about the prescriber etc.

'Well, I am still going to get to the bottom of this with Sally and whoever prescribed this.'

OSCE Answer sheet (for OSCE 6.3)

Candidate name:		Date:	

You will not need to submit this page for assessment.

Date:
Issue details:

Final Outcome:

👥 Buddy activity

Example 6.4 OSCE Station – Dealing with an ethical dilemma

Please read the following information carefully. You have 10 minutes to complete the task

Background

You are a pharmacist prescriber working in an oncology department. You have a new patient, Mr Lockwood (70 years old).

History

Mr Lockwood has pancreatic cancer which is inoperable and he is terminally ill. Mr Lockwood is aware that he has a form of cancer but as yet has not been told his prognosis. He will be offered treatment but it is palliative only. The nurse on the ward is concerned that he will not be able to cope with the news.

Mr Lockwood has been treated for anxiety and depression in the past.

Task

1. Discuss the issue appropriately with the nurse.

2. Document the interaction on the resource provided. You are assessed on what you **say** to the **other healthcare professional**.

You are provided with sources for the discussion, including the healthcare professional. There are two people seated at the station; the examiner and healthcare professional. Introduce yourself to the patient when you are ready to begin.

Please submit your answer sheet to the examiner at the end of the OSCE and do not forget to include your name on the form.

DO NOT write on or remove the patient information leaflet or any other materials provided.

Station props that would be provided

Item required

1. Instructions for candidate.

2. Candidate answer sheet.

3. Script for Elizabeth Emery (nurse actor).

4. Mark sheet.

5. RPS Medicines, Ethics and Practice Guide – http://www.rpharms.com/support/mep.asp.

OSCE (ethical dilemma) – Script for actor (OSCE 6.4)

You are Elizabeth Emery, a 22-year-old registered nurse who has just joined the oncology department.

You are very concerned about your patient Mr Lockwood.

Mr Lockwood has pancreatic cancer which is inoperable and he is terminally ill. Mr Lockwood is aware that he has a form of cancer but as yet has not been told his prognosis. Mr Lockwood lives independently and has no immediate family for support. You feel that he is an extremely anxious individual.

After a number of conversations with the patient you are concerned that he will not be able to cope with the news and you have asked one of the senior pharmacists to persuade the rest of the team to withhold the prognosis.

If the candidate asks about the nature of query/issue, say...

'I am concerned that Mr Lockwood will not be able to handle the news. Could you persuade the rest of the team to not tell him at this point that he has this death sentence hanging over his head? You're a senior person, they will listen to you.'

If the candidate asks why you feel this way, say...

'I have had a number of conversations with Mr Lockwood, he has no family and seems so anxious. He seems to have a history of anxiety and panic attacks. He will simply not be able to cope with this news.'

If the candidate asks about what the patient does know at this stage, say...

'He knows he has cancer but we don't need to tell him that the treatment is palliative. We are not lying by doing this!'

The conversation can be closed with...

If the candidate refuses to discuss this issue with the team with no explanation, say...

'What happened to putting the patient first?'

If the candidate explains the reasons why truth telling is important say,

'OK, I can see where you are coming from. We can work with the rest of team to get him some support.'

OSCE Candidate notes page (for OSCE 6.4)

Candidate name:		Date:	

You will not need to submit this page for assessment.

Date:
Issue details:

Final Outcome:

OSCE station mark sheet (for OSCE 6.1)

Candidate's Name		Date	

Assessment criteria		Mark	
Communication points:			
1. Introduce themselves including name **(1 mark)** and position **(1 mark)**	0	1	2
2. Asks to speak to the prescriber by the *correct* name **(1 mark)**	0	1	-
3. Explains reason for query **(1 mark)** and specifies patient (including unique identifier) **(1 mark)**	0	1	2
4. Candidate closes conversation appropriately i.e. thanks doctor for his/her time etc.	0	1	-
Knowledge points:			
Issue 1: Methotrexate is prescribed daily			
5. Identifies that methotrexate is prescribed daily instead of weekly on a Tuesday	0	-	2
6. ***Candidate should explicitly ask doctor to amend the prescription to weekly and on a Tuesday***	0	-	2
Issue 2: Folic acid is prescribed daily			
7. Identifies that folic acid is prescribed daily instead of weekly	0	1	-
8. Recognises that folic acid is not recommended to be taken on the same day as methotrexate **(1 mark)** due to opposition of folate antagonism **(1 mark)**	0	1	2
9. Ask doctor to change frequency to be taken to once a week on Thursday as per pre-admission schedule **(1 mark)**	0	1	-
Issue 3: Ibuprofen interacts with methotrexate			
10. Ibuprofen interacts with methotrexate to increase toxicity **(1 mark)**	0	1	-
11. Candidate should suggest appropriate alternative NSAID **(1 mark)** if requested to do so	0	1	-
DISCRETIONARYAny other valid point up to a maximum of 2 marks e.g.			
12. Monitoring FBC/LFT/RF with methotrexate	0	1	2
13. Monitoring RF/Hb with NSAIDS			
14. Monitoring pain score			
15. Complete an incident form			
16. Other (please state)			

Communication style:		
Excellent	All of the time: appropriately assertive with doctor; correct recommendations are made; body language appropriate & eye contact good.	4
Good	Most of the time: appropriately assertive with doctor; correct recommendations are made; body language appropriate & eye contact good.	3
Average	Some of the time: appropriately assertive with doctor; correct recommendations are made; body language appropriate & eye contact good.	2

Continued

OSCE station mark sheet (for OSCE 6.1)—cont'd

Poor	Most of the time: inappropriately assertive with doctor; incorrect recommendations are made; body language inappropriate & eye contact poor.	1
Fail	All of the time: inappropriately assertive with doctor; incorrect recommendations are made; body language inappropriate & eye contact poor.	0

Issue(s) relating to patient safety:

If candidates propose any course of action which could lead to serious harm or death, they will **fail** the OSCE. Always seek a second opinion. Give detail:

Total Mark:	/20 (max)	
Angoff score: 11 Criterion in bold italics is essential (criterion 6)	**Pass**	**Fail**

OSCE station mark sheet (for OSCE 6.2)

Candidate's Name		Date	

Assessment criteria	Mark		
Communication points:			
1. Introduces themselves including name **(1 mark)** and position **(1 mark)**	0	1	2
2. Asks to speak to the prescriber by the *correct* name **(1 mark)**	0	1	-
3. Explains reason for query **(1 mark)** and specifies patient (including unique identifier) **(1 mark)**	0	1	2
4. Candidate closes conversation appropriately i.e. thanks doctor for his/her time etc.	0	1	-
Knowledge points:			
Issue 1: Candesartan is unsafe in pregnancy and should not be prescribed			
5. Identifies that candesartan is contra-indicated/is unsafe to prescribe in pregnancy	0	-	2
6. Candidate should specify that candesartan can cause foetal or neonatal problems with blood flow, renal function and skull defects	0	1	-
7. *Candidate should explicitly ask doctor to stop the prescription for the candesartan OR switch/change the candesartan to a reasonably safe alternative*	0	-	2
8. Candidate should suggest a reasonably safe alternative (e.g. methyldopa, labetalol, nifedipine)	0	-	2
Issue 2: Diprobase is omitted from the kardex			
9. Identifies that Diprobase is omitted from the kardex	0	-	2
10. Candidate should explicitly ask doctor to prescribe Diprobase cream on the kardex **(1 mark)**, recommending the correct dose frequency – i.e. apply to hands twice a day **(1 mark)**	0	1	2

OSCE station mark sheet (for OSCE 6.2)—cont'd

DISCRETIONARYAny other valid point up to a maximum of 2 marks e.g.

	0	1	2
11. Monitor blood pressure			
12. Monitor pain score			
13. Complete an incident form			
14. Other (please state)			

Communication style:

Excellent	All of the time: appropriately assertive with doctor; correct recommendations are made; body language appropriate & eye contact good.	4
Good	Most of the time: appropriately assertive with doctor; correct recommendations are made; body language appropriate & eye contact good.	3
Average	Some of the time: appropriately assertive with doctor; correct recommendations are made; body language appropriate & eye contact good.	2
Poor	Most of the time: inappropriately assertive with doctor; incorrect recommendations are made; body language inappropriate & eye contact poor.	1
Fail	All of the time: inappropriately assertive with doctor; incorrect recommendations are made; body language inappropriate & eye contact poor.	0

Issue(s) relating to patient safety:

If candidates propose any course of action which could lead to serious harm or death, they will **fail** the OSCE. Always seek a second opinion. Give detail:

Total Mark:	/21	
Angoff score: 10 Criterion in bold italics is essential (criterion 7)	Pass	Fail

Assessor's comments:

Assessor's Signature:_____

OSCE station mark sheet (for OSCE 6.3)

Candidate's Name		Date	

Assessment criteria	Mark		
Communication points:			
1. Introduce themselves including name **(1 mark)** and position **(1 mark)**	0	1	2
2. Asks/allows Mrs Finbar to explain the query **(1 mark)**	0	1	-
3. Establishes that the patient is Sally Finbar **(1 mark)** and that she is not present **(1 mark)**	0	1	2
4. Establishes the age of the patient	0	1	
5. Establishes that the patient is unaware of this discussion	0	1	
6. Establishes that Sally does not belong to a vulnerable group	0	1	
7. Acknowledges that this is an upsetting situation for the parent	0	1	
8. Candidate closes conversation appropriately	0	1	-
Knowledge and reasoning points:			
Issue: Confidentiality			
9. **Explains to the parent that as the patient is not present the information cannot be discussed**	0	-	2
10. Explains general duty of confidentiality which applies	0		2
11. Explains the general guidance on prescribing contraceptives	0		2
12. Suggests an open discussion between Mrs Finbar and Sally as a way forward	0	-	2
DISCRETIONARYAny other valid point up to a maximum of 2 marks e.g.			
13. Refers patient to appropriate guidance on confidentiality (MEP p 141)	0	1	2
14. Other (please state)			

Communication style:		
Excellent	**All of the time:** appropriate approach with parent; correct recommendations are made; body language appropriate & eye contact good.	4
Good	**Most of the time:** appropriate approach with parent; correct recommendations are made; body language appropriate & eye contact good.	3
Average	**Some of the time:** appropriate approach with parent; correct recommendations are made; body language appropriate & eye contact good.	2
Poor	**Most of the time:** appropriate approach with parent; incorrect recommendations are made; body language inappropriate & eye contact poor.	1
Fail	**All of the time:** appropriate approach with parent; incorrect recommendations are made; body language inappropriate & eye contact poor.	0

Issue(s) relating to patient safety:

If candidates propose any course of action which could lead to serious harm or death, they will **fail** the OSCE. Always seek a second opinion. Give detail:

OSCE station mark sheet (for OSCE 6.3)—cont'd

Total Mark:		/22	
Angoff score: 9 Criterion in bold italics is essential (criterion 9)		Pass	Fail

Assessor's comments:

Assessor's Signature:_____

OSCE station mark sheet (for OSCE 6.4)

Candidate's Name		Date	

Assessment criteria	Mark		
Communication points:			
1. Asks/allows Elizabeth Emery to explain the query/issue **(1 mark)**	0	1	-
2. Establishes the reason for concern, living alone **(1 mark)** history of anxiety **(1 mark)**	0	1	2
3. Acknowledge the nurse's role as patient advocate	0	1	
4. Candidate closes conversation appropriately	0	1	-
Knowledge and reasoning points:			
Issue: Truth telling			
5. *Explains that patients need to be fully informed for the purpose of autonomy/ right to know/consent (or similar wording)*	0	-	2
6. Explains that the patient will know something is wrong	0	1	
7. Explains that Mr Lockwood may lose trust in the team if he finds out the full details at a later date	0	1	
8. Explains that the team cannot withhold information	0	1	
9. Suggests that the patient may wish to put his affairs in order if limited time is left	0	1	
10. Suggests further discussion with the team to voice concerns and establish a support network for the patient	0		2
DISCRETIONARYAny other valid point up to a maximum of 2 marks e.g.			
11. Refers nurse to appropriate guidance on consent	0	1	2
12. Other (please state)			

Continued

OSCE station mark sheet (for OSCE 6.4)—cont'd

Communication style:

Excellent	**All of the time:** appropriate approach with parent; correct recommendations are made; body language appropriate & eye contact good.	4
Good	**Most of the time:** appropriate approach with parent; correct recommendations are made; body language appropriate & eye contact good.	3
Average	**Some of the time:** appropriate approach with parent; correct recommendations are made; body language appropriate & eye contact good.	2
Poor	**Most of the time:** appropriate approach with parent; incorrect recommendations are made; body language inappropriate & eye contact poor.	1
Fail	**All of the time:** appropriate approach with parent; incorrect recommendations are made; body language inappropriate & eye contact poor.	0

Issue(s) relating to patient safety:

If candidates propose any course of action which could lead to serious harm or death, they will **fail** the OSCE. Always seek a second opinion. Give detail:

Total Mark:		/17	
Angoff score: 7 Criterion in bold italics is essential (criterion 5)		**Pass**	**Fail**

Assessor's comments:

Assessor's Signature:_____

✔ How to excel in this type of station

Action	Reason	How
Be systematic	If you are e.g. reviewing the medication chart / kardex. Always also look to see if the medication has been given to the patient i.e. has a nurse signed the administration section so you can judge how to act if the patient has actually received the medication or not.	Start at the first page and look at the patient details including allergy status and then move on to the medications prescribed regularly, when required and as once only – checking their doses, frequencies etc.
Self-check any recommendations	It is easy to make an error when reading information from an unfamiliar monograph or guideline, take your time.	If you are e.g. recommending a dose increase or reduction or a change of medication, check your information at least twice to ensure you have documented this clearly for the prescriber.
Self-check any calculations	Dosing errors can lead to non-improvement from under-dose or patient harm if an overdose particularly in extremes of age or weight, particularly if the medication is one with which you are unfamiliar.	If you are familiar with the medication, consider what you think is a reasonable dose for this individual patient; this will help you judge if your calculation appears plausible. For example, if you calculate the rate of a dopamine infusion to be 1,000 ml/hr, is this reasonable? Can this be given to a patient?
Interacting professionally with the Dr at the station	Professional behaviour is essential and appropriately assertive communication skills are vital to ensuring you have a successful interaction with the Doctor present; ensure you know their name and also that you have all of your information at hand when you speak to them.	When asking e.g. Dr Jones if you can speak to them about a patient, remember to explain which patient it is clearly. Always start with the most important issue first and provide a resolution to all issues identified. If you have second or third issue to address, it may be useful to start the conversation by saying "I have a number of issues to discuss with but the most important is…" to ensure that you address all of the identified problems in the timeframe. Refer to the props e.g. the medication chart or other information at the station to enhance your interaction and make your points more clearly.

Further reading

Beauchamp, T., Childress, J., 1994. Principles of biomedical ethics, 4th ed. Oxford University Press, New York, p. 11.

Braunack-Mayer, A., 2001. What makes a problem an ethical problem? An empirical perspective on the nature of ethical problems in general practice. J. Med. Ethics 27, 98–103.

Bridges, D.R., Davidson, R.A., Odegard, P.S., et al., 2011. Interprofessional collaboration: three best practice models of interprofessional education. Med. Educ. Online 16.

Centre for the Advancement of Interprofessional Education (CAIPE), Retrieved on 18 August 2015 from <www.caipe.org.uk>.

Cooper, R.J., Bissell, P., Wingfield, J., 2008. Ethical decision-making, passivity and pharmacy. J. Med. Ethics 34, 441–445.

General Pharmaceutical Council, GPhC Code of Ethics. Retrieved on 14 October 2015 from <https://www.pharmacyregulation.org/sites/default/files/standards_of_conduct_ethics_and_performance_july_2014.pdf>.

Lo, B., 2013. Resolving ethical dilemmas: a guide for clinicians, 5th ed. Wolters Kluwer Health, Philadelphia.

Pharmaceutical Society of Northern Ireland, PSNI Code of Ethics. Retrieved on October 14, 2015 from <http://www.psni.org.uk/documents/312/Code+of+Ethics+for+Pharmacists+in+Northern+Ireland.pdf>.

Royal Pharmaceutical Society, Medicines, Ethics and Practice guide 39. Retrieved on 14 October 2015 from <http://www.rpharms.com/support/mep.asp>.

Zillich, A.J., McDonough, P., Carter, B.L., Doucette, W.R., 2004. Influential characteristics of physician/pharmacist collaborative relationships. Ann. Pharmacother. 38, 764–770.

Background

Prescribing rights have extended to a number of healthcare professionals with the implementation of recommendations from the Crown Report in 1989. Non-medical prescribing aims to give patients quicker access to medicines, improve access to services and make better use of nurses, pharmacists and other healthcare professionals' skills. Currently pharmacists in the UK can only prescribe after successfully completing an accredited course two years post qualification and must have their names annotated on the General Pharmaceutical Council (GPhC) or Pharmaceutical Society of Northern Ireland (PSNI) registry. However, many MPharm courses in the UK offer foundational modules or learning in prescribing and medicines optimisation/pharmaceutical care; therefore you will be developing prescribing skills for further advancement once qualified. The Royal Pharmaceutical Society published a competency framework for all prescribers in 2016 (see Figure 7.1). Some of the key skills

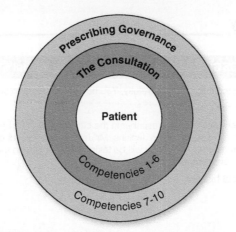

The Consultation	Prescribing Governance
1. Assess the patient	7. Prescribe safely
2. Consider the options	8. Prescribe professionally
3. Reach a shared decision	9. Improve prescribing practice
4. Prescribe	10. Prescribe as part of a team
5. Provide information	
6. Monitor and review	

Figure 7.1 RPS Competency framework for all prescribers.

and competencies that you may develop during your undergraduate course include the following.

The pharmacy student:

- Identifies, accesses, and uses reliable and validated sources of information and critically evaluates other information.
- Explores the patient/carers understanding of a consultation and aims for a satisfactory outcome for the patient/carer and prescriber.
- Understands the potential for adverse effects and takes steps to avoid/minimise, recognise and manage them.
- Makes accurate legible and contemporaneous records and clinical notes of prescribing decisions.

(From the RPS: A Competency Framework for all Prescribers, July 2016.)

Preparation

In this chapter two prescribing OSCE stations are presented, a verbal and a written station. Once again you should check that your course has covered the topics and competencies before attempting the station. Most prescribing skills are taught in the final year of the MPharm and therefore these may be too advanced for level 1 or 2 students. Your course provider may use local formularies and guidelines for prescribing and it would be useful to refer to these where appropriate.

👥 Buddy Activity

Example 7.1.   OSCE Examination – Prescribing Verbal Station

Please read the following information carefully. You have 10 minutes to complete the task.

Background

You are an independent pharmacist prescriber in the city hospital. You have taken on a case load of patients this week which includes Robin Jenkins. Mr Jenkins is 55 years old, suffers from COPD and was diagnosed 6 months ago. Today you will be taking over his care in the respiratory clinic as an independent pharmacist prescriber.

Past medical/surgical history

DOB: 06.01.59

COPD

Ex-smoker

FEV₁ 53% predicted

Current medication

Asmasal Clickhaler® (salbutamol 95 µg/metered inhalation) 1 or 2 puffs when required

Paracetamol tablets 500 mg 1 or 2 tablets when required (max 8 daily)

The task below is part of your initial consultation with the patient.

Example 7.1. OSCE Examination – Prescribing Verbal Station—cont'd

Task

As a prescriber, you have decided to add a long-acting muscarinic antagonist to his current medication regimen as his current inhaler is not helping with his breathlessness. You have decided to prescribe Spiriva® capsules with a HandiHaler®.

1. Introduce yourself as the pharmacist prescriber and explain that you will be prescribing for Mr Jenkins in your clinic.

2. Decide on an initial dose and counsel him on the appropriate usage using the inhaler and PIL provided.

3. Complete your consultation document for the medical records

You are provided with resources for the consultation, including the patient. The station demonstrator will play the part of the patient – let the supervisor know when you are ready to speak with him or her.

Please submit your answer sheet to the examiner at the end of the OSCE and do not forget to include your name on the form.

DO NOT write on or remove any materials provided

Station props that would be provided

Items required

1. Instructions for candidate.

2. Copy of instructions for examiner (observer).

3. Copy of instructions and script for patient actor.

4. Candidate answer sheet (consultation record).

5. Examiner's mark sheet.

6. Inhaler and PIL.

OSCE Prescribing Verbal Station – Notes to patient actor (for OSCE 7.1)

The candidate is playing the role of the pharmacist prescriber. You are Robin Jenkins and you suffer from a lung disease known as chronic obstructive pulmonary disease or COPD (diagnosis made 6 months ago). This condition leaves you short of breath and vulnerable to chest infections.

You already use a dry powdered inhaler called Asmasal® Clickhaler® which you know contains salbutamol. The Clickhaler® is not as good as it used to be and you are finding that you are using it several times a day and sometimes a lot more every day. You are aware that as the condition progresses they will need to add on inhalers.

DOB 06.01.59, a retired engineer, married with 3 grown-up children.

You attend the respiratory clinic in the city hospital every 6 months. Today you will meet a new pharmacist who is qualified to prescribe and will take over your care in his or her clinic.

You have been prescribed a new inhaler and the student must complete the following tasks with you:

Student task

1. Introduce yourself as the pharmacist prescriber and explain that you will be prescribing for Mr Jenkins in your clinic.

2. You have decided to prescribe Spiriva® capsules with a HandiHaler® and you must decide on an initial dose and counsel him on the appropriate usage using the inhaler and PIL provided.

3. Complete your consultation document for the medical records.

OSCE Prescribing Verbal Station – Script for patient actor (for OSCE 7.1)

If the candidate does not identify you, say...

'Are you sure that you are talking to the right person? I would not want you to mix me up with someone else.'

If the candidate asks your date of birth, address or weight, say...

06.01.59

27 Garland Drive

Belfast

If the candidate asks if you know what kind of inhaler you have been prescribed you can say...

'No, I am not entirely sure. What kind is it?'

The candidate will then demonstrate the use of the inhaler – listen carefully and if the candidate asks you, you can repeat the instructions.

You should ask the candidate...

'Am I going to still use the Asmasal® Clickhaler® when I need to?'

The answer to this should be yes! If the candidate says no you should agree to this.

If the candidate asks if you are concordant/adherent with your medicines, say...

'I'm not sure what you mean...?'

If the candidate asks if you remember to use your medicines as prescribed, say...

'Oh yes, I am very careful with my inhaler but I found that the Clickhaler® just wasn't enough...'

If the candidate asks you if you have any questions you would like to ask, say...

'No thanks, I think you have told me all that I need to know.'

OSCE Prescribing Verbal Station – Consultation Notes (for OSCE 7.1)

Candidate name:		Date:	

Use the space below to record your consultation notes.

Patient details
Patient name: Mr Robin Jenkins
Patient address: 27 Garland Drive, Belfast
DOB: 06.01.59
Patient Number: CH 99/03620

Consultation notes:

Date and time of consultation:

Medication prescribed:

Dose:

Side effects discussed :

Other advice:

Signature _____

Role_____

GPhC Competencies for station 7.1	Level 4
10.2.2 (g) Communicate with patients about their prescribed treatment	– shows how
10.2.2 (i) Record, maintain and store patient data	– shows how
10.2.4 (f) Conclude consultation to ensure a satisfactory outcome	– shows how
10.2.4 (g) Maintain accurate and comprehensive consultation records	– shows how
10.2.4 (h) Provide accurate written or oral information appropriate to the needs of patients, the public or other healthcare professionals	– shows how
10.2.5 (a) demonstrate the characteristics of a prospective professional pharmacist as set out in relevant codes of conduct and behaviour	– does

OSCE Examination: Example 7.2 – Prescribing Written

Background

You are an independent pharmacist prescriber in the city hospital. Mr Pinstone attends a diabetes clinic following his diagnosis in 2010 (type 1 diabetes). Today you will be taking over his care in the clinic as an independent pharmacist prescriber.

Past medical/surgical history

Mr Pinstone self-administers NovoRapid® (12 units in the morning, 10 units at lunchtime and 8 units at teatime) and Lantus® at night (18 units). Mr Pinstone's blood lipid profile and liver function test have come back from the laboratory with a high cholesterol profile and a statin must be initiated. Mr Pinstone has no known drug allergies.

Task

1. Prescribe an appropriate statin on the kardex provided.

2. Record in the clinical notes the lipid profile results and further laboratory tests, if required.

3. Record in the clinical notes the counselling points that need to be discussed with the patient.

Please submit your answer sheet to the examiner at the end of the OSCE and do not forget to include your name on the form.

DO NOT write on or remove any materials provided.

Station props that would be provided

Items required

1. Instructions for candidate.

2. Copy of instructions for examiner (observer).

3. Candidate answer sheet (clinical notes).

4. Mark sheet.

5. BNF.

6. Kardex for David Pinstone (Fig. 7.2).

7. Local guidelines on statins (based on 2014 NICE guidelines 181).

8. Clinical laboratory results for patient

OSCE Prescribing Written Station – Clinical Notes (for OSCE 7.2)

Candidate name:		Date:	

Use the space below to record your clinical notes.

Patient details
Patient name: Mr David Pinstone
Patient address: 11 Sycamore Street, Belfast
DOB: 11.3.78

Clinical notes

Date and time:

Results:

Prescribing details:

Counselling points:

Labs requested:

Signature _____

Role_____

	WQA7000 Rev. October 2011

Medicine Prescription and Administration Record

Rewritten on (date):

Record: of

Allergies / Medicine Sensitivities

THIS SECTION **MUST** BE COMPLETED

Date	Medicine (generic) / Allergen	Type of Reaction	Signature

OR

No Known allergies ☑ Please tick

Signature: C.Jones   Date: x/xx/xx

Write in CAPITAL LETTERS or use addressograph

Surname: Pinstone

First Names: David

Hospital No: 1456789

DOB: 11/3/78   *Check identity*

Hospital: The Trust   Ward: West Four

Consultant: Jones

Date of Admission: x/xx/xx

Admissions Medicines Reconciliation completed

Sign: .... Date: ....

Discharge prescription ordered by

Sign: .... Date: ....

Weight (Kg)	Date	Height (cm)
60kg		173 cm

Requirements for Prescribing and Administration

- Nurses must not administer medicines that are improperly or illegibly prescribed.
- Do not prescribe or administer medication if the allergy status is not documented and signed (unless in an emergency).
- Prescribe generically (refer to WHSCT Policy for appropriate use of approved/generic names of medicines).
- Print the full name of the medicine in CAPITALS in black ink. Do not abbreviate medicine names.
- Do not alter existing instructions. Cancel and rewrite any changes in medicine therapy.
- Discontinue any therapy by drawing a diagonal line through the prescription and the remainder of the administration record. Enter the date of discontinuation and signature in the 'Stop' space.
- Do not abbreviate 'micrograms', 'nanograms', 'international units' or units; write in full.
- Prescriber's signatures must be written in full; initials are not acceptable.
- Other prescriptions in use must be referenced on the main prescription record.
- Attach all additional charts to the Medicine Prescription and Administration record.
- The administering nurse(s) must initial each administration.
- All kardexes must be rewritten after 14 days.
- Medicines reconciliation - for each regular or when required medicine, indicate changes made to therapy during stay.
  - On admission, refer to the patient's documented medication history, reconcile medicines on the kardex and circle 'no change', 'increased dose', 'decreased dose' or 'new' medicine accordingly.
  - During patient stay, ensure any subsequent changes are similarly indicated and document the reason in the table below.
  - At discharge, ensure information on medicine changes (including stopped medication) is sent to the GP.

Additional Charts in Use *(please tick)*

Epidural ☐	Intrathecal ☐	Blood Sugar Monitoring ☐	Total Parenteral Nutrition (TPN) ☐	Other (please specify) ☐
Patient Controlled Analgesia ☐	Diabetic Ketoacidosis ☐	Fluid Balance ☐	Oral Anticoagulant ☐	Syringe Driver (please indicate 1 or more) ☐
Insulin ☐	Chemotherapy ☐	Anaesthetic Record ☐	Endoscopy ☐	

Special Instructions / Additional Notes on Medicines / Reason for Medicine Omission *(please sign and date)*

Medicines Reconciliation Record During Patient's Stay

	Medication	Commenced in Hospital (tick if YES)	Stopped in Hospital (tick if YES)	Dose Changed ↑ or ↓	Reason for Medication Change
1					
2					
3					
4					
5					

1   OS17629

Figure 7.2 Student kardex for completion (for OSCE 7.2).

Venous Thromboembolism (VTE) Risk Assessment for Hospitalised Adults

Risk assessment must be completed on admission

Write in CAPITAL LETTERS or use addressograph

Surname: ....

First Names: ....

Hospital No: ....

DOB: .... *Check identity*

Step 1: Assess for level of mobility – All Patients

	Tick		Tick		Tick
Surgical patient		Medical patient expected to have ongoing reduced mobility relative to normal state		Medical patient NOT expected to have significantly reduced mobility relative to normal state	
		Assess for thrombosis and bleeding risk below (Complete steps 2 – 5)		Risk assessment complete (Go to step 5)⊠	

Step 2: Review thrombosis risk

Any tick for thrombosis risk factors should prompt consideration for thromboprophylaxis

Patient related	Tick	Admission related	Tick
Active cancer or cancer treatment		Significantly reduced mobility for 3 days or more	
Age >60		Hip or knee replacement	
Dehydration		Hip fracture	
Known thrombophilias		Total anaesthetic + surgery time > 90 minutes	
Personal history / first degree relative with history of VTE		Surgery involving pelvis or lower limb with anaesthetic + surgery time > 60 minutes	
One or more significant medical comorbidities (eg heart disease; metabolic, endocrine or respiratory pathologies; acute infectious diseases; inflammatory conditions)		Acute surgical admission with inflammatory or intra-abdominal condition	
Obesity (BMI>30kg/m^2)		Critical care admission	
Use of hormone replacement therapy		Surgery with significant reduction in mobility	
Use of oestrogen-containing oral contraceptive therapy		**The above risk factors are not exhaustive, additional risks may be considered. Other:**	
Varicose veins with phlebitis			
Pregnancy or < 6 weeks post partum (see obstetric risk assessment for VTE)			

Step 3: Review bleeding risk

Any tick should prompt staff to consider if bleeding risk is sufficient to preclude pharmacological intervention

Patient related	Tick	Admission related	Tick
Active bleeding		Neurosurgery, spinal surgery or eye surgery	
Acquired bleeding disorder (such as acute liver failure)		Lumbar puncture / epidural / spinal anaesthesia expected in the next 12 hours	
Concurrent use of anticoagulants known to increase risk of bleeding (such as warfarin with INR >2)		Lumbar puncture / epidural / spinal anaesthesia within the previous 4 hours	
Acute stroke		Other procedure with high bleeding risk	
Thrombocytopaenia (Platelets <75x10^9/l)		**The above risk factors are not exhaustive, additional risks may be considered. Other:**	
Uncontrolled systolic hypertension (>230/120)			
Untreated inherited bleeding disorder (such as haemophilia and von Willebrand's disease)			

Step 4: Tick the appropriate risk category

Risk of VTE (tick)	High risk of VTE with low bleeding risk		High risk of VTE with significant bleeding risk		Low risk of VTE	
Thromboprophylaxis prescribed on kardex? (tick)	Yes		Type Prescribed (tick)	Pharmacological e.g. LMWH		
	No			Mechanical		

Step 5: Signature

VTE risk assessed on admission	Signature:	Print Name:	Date and Time:

VTE risk should be re-assessed within 24 hours and whenever clinical condition changes

Northern Ireland VTE Advisory Group, June 2011

Figure 7.2—cont'd

Continued

Once Only Medicines and Pre-Medications
(includes administration under Patient Group Direction)

If more than one Kardex, ensure 'once only' medicines are written on
'1 of 2' Kardex, until once only section on that Kardex is complete.

Patient Name: ....

Hospital Number: ....
(complete if photocopying page)

Prescription						Administration		
Date	Medicine	Dose	Route	Time to be given (24 hour clock)	Signature	Given by	Time given (24 hour clock)	Pharmacy

Figure 7.2—cont'd

Regular Non-Injectable Medication
Check allergy status and patient identity

Codes for recording omitted doses

ⓃN = nil by mouth   ⓋV = vomiting
ⓇR = patient refused   ⒹD = drug not available
ⓅP = patient not available   ⓄO = other*
ⓈS = unable to swallow   PRⓇPrescribed omission*
*Record reasons in medical/nursing notes.

Take action on omitted doses as appropriate

Write in CAPITAL LETTERS or use addressograph

Surname: ....
First Names: ....
Consultant: .... Ward: ....
Hospital No: ....
D.O.B: .... *Check identity*

Year:				Day and Month: →														
Circle times or enter variable dose/time				▼ ▼														
Medicine				06⁰⁰														
Dose		Route	Start Date	Stop Date	08⁰⁰													
Special Instructions/Directions				Signature	12⁰⁰													
					14⁰⁰													
Medicines Reconciliation (circle)					18⁰⁰													
No Change	Increased Dose	Decreased Dose	New															
Signature	Print Name			Pharmacy	22⁰⁰													
Bleep																		

(The structure above — Medicine block with times 06:00, 08:00, 12:00, 14:00, 18:00, 22:00 and Medicines Reconciliation rows — repeats five times down the chart.)

5

City Hospital

Out-patients

CH 123456
PINSTONE
DAVID
111 SYCAMORE STEET 11/03/78

CON DOBSON WARD B1

Sample received: yesterday's date

Lipid Profile

SERUM	OBSERVED VALUE	REFERENCE INTERVAL
Triglycerides	*1.78mmol/L	(0.3–1.7)
Cholesterol	*8.8mmol/L	(0.5–5.0)
HDL- cholesterol	1.0mmol/L	(1.0–2.7)
LDL	*3.9mmol/L	(0.1–3.0)
Chol/HDL Ratio	*8.8	(0–5.0)

Date of specimen: yesterday's date

Lab. ACC. No.: 1146 DS

Dr T Reid, Consultant Pathologist
City Hospital Clinical Chemistry Lab

Liver Function Tests

Serum interval	OBSERVED VALUE	REFERENCE
Total bilirubin	12umol/L	(3–17)
Alk, Phosphatase (ALP)	58U/L	(35–120)
Aspartate Aminotransferase	21U/L	(10–40)
Gammaglutamyl transferas	23U/L	(12–58)
Albumin	36g/L	(35–50)

Figure 7.3 Clinical laboratory results for David Pinstone.

GPhC Competencies for station 7.2	Level 4
10.2.1 (b) access and critically evaluate evidence to support safe, rational and cost-effective use of medicines	– shows how
10.2.2 (e) clinically evaluate the appropriateness of prescribed medicines	– shows how
10.2.2 (f) provide, monitor and modify prescribed treatment to maximise health outcomes	– shows how
10.2.4 (g) Maintain accurate and comprehensive consultation records	– shows how
10.2.2 (i) Record, maintain and store patient data – shows how	– shows how

OSCE station mark sheet (for OSCE 7.1)

Candidate's Name		Date		

Assessment criteria:	Mark			
1. Introduce themselves including name **(1 mark)** and role **(1 mark)**	0	1	2	-
2. Identifies that this is the correct patient using name and one other unique identifier.	0	1	-	-
3. Explains the purpose of the discussion	0	1	-	-
4. Explains to the patient that he must inhale one capsule daily (18 µg)	0	-	2	
5a. To release the dust cap press the piercing button completely in and let go.	0	1		
b. Open the dust cap completely by pulling it upwards. Then open the mouthpiece by pulling it upwards.	0	1		
c. Remove a SPIRIVA capsule from the blister (only immediately before use, see blister handling) and place it in the centre chamber.	0	1		
d. Close the mouthpiece firmly until you hear a click, leaving the dust cap open.	0	1		
e. Hold the HandiHaler® device with the mouthpiece upwards and press the piercing button completely in only once, and release. This makes holes in the capsule and allows the medication to be released when you breathe in.	0	1		
f. Breathe out completely.	0	1		
g. Raise the HandiHaler® to your mouth and close your lips tightly around the mouthpiece.	0	1		
h. Keep your head in an upright position and breathe in slowly and deeply but at a rate sufficient to hear or feel the capsule vibrate.	0	1		
i. Breathe until your lungs are full; then hold your breath as long as comfortable and at the same time take the HandiHaler® out of your mouth.	0	1		
j. Resume normal breathing. Repeat steps f and g once, in order to empty the capsule completely.	0	1		
k. Open the mouthpiece again. Tip out the used capsule and dispose. Close the mouthpiece and dust cap for storage of your HandiHaler® device.	0	1		
6. Discusses side effects with patient e.g. dry mouth	0	1		-
7. Documents				

Continued

OSCE station mark sheet (for OSCE 7.1)—cont'd

	0	1	
Date and time of consultation	0	1	
Medication prescribed	0	1	
Dose	0	1	
Side effects	0	1	
Any other advice given	0	1	
Signature **(1 mark)**, role **(1 mark)**	0	1	2
8. Asks patient if he has any questions and answers correctly	0	1	-	-
9. If the student uses inappropriate language or does not use suitable layman's terms	-1			
10. Thanks the patient for his time	0	1	-	-

Issue(s) relating to patient safety

11. If candidates proposes any course of action which could lead to serious harm or death, they will **fail** the OSCE. Always seek a second opinion. Give detail:

Professionalism including communication style

Excellent	**All of the time:** appropriately attentive; empathetic and interested; identifies and resolves health promotion issues; doesn't cause embarrassment or loss of face; checks understanding; organised questioning; body language appropriate & eye contact good.	4
Good	**Most of the time** (as above).	3
Average	**Some of the time** (as above).	2
Poor	**Most of the time:** inattentive; lack of empathy and interest; does not identify or resolve health promotion issues; causes embarrassment or loss of face; does not check understanding; disorganised questioning; body language inappropriate & eye contact poor.	1
Fail	**All of the time:** (as above).	0

If the candidate proposes any course of action which could lead to serious harm or death, they will **fail** the OSCE. Always seek a second opinion. Give detail: _____

Total Mark (31 marks)	**/31**	
Angoff score (borderline competence): 14	Pass	Fail
Criterion in bold italics is essential (criterion 4)		

Assessor's comments:

Assessor's signature_____

OSCE station mark sheet (for OSCE 7.2)

Candidate's Name		Date		

Assessment criteria:	Mark		
1. Prescribes a statin correctly using the kardex; local formulary recommends atorvastatin 20 mg or suitable alternative from BNF (all in bold are essential) **Name** **Strength** **Frequency** **Signs the kardex** **Dates the kardex**	0	-	2
Form	0	1	
2. Clinical notes			
Date	0	1	
Time	0	1	
Lipid profile results recorded correctly (ref range not required)	0	1	
What was prescribed (name, strength and frequency)	0	1	
Counselling points – reporting unexplained muscle weakness, pain or tenderness	0	1	
Laboratory test recorded — LFTs within 3 months **(1 mark)** and 12 months **(1 mark)**	0	1	2
Signature **(1 mark)**, role **(1 mark)**	0	1	2
Issue(s) relating to patient safety			
3. If candidates propose any course of action which could lead to serious harm or death, they will fail the OSCE. Always seek a second opinion. Give detail:			

Total Mark (12 marks)	/12	
Angoff score (borderline competence): 6 Criterion in bold italics is essential (criterion 1)	Pass	Fail

Assessor's comments:

Assessor's signature_____

✔ **How to excel in this type of station**

Action	Reason	How
Checking understanding and details	When prescribing it is important to double check that your patient has understood the information. Are they happy with what has been prescribed and why?	Ask the patient to repeat your instructions. Check their understanding and leave time at the end to answer their questions.

✘ **Common errors in this type of station**

Action	Remedy	Reason
Incorrect details	Check dates, directions and signatures when prescribing on a kardex or a community prescription.	If dates etc. are incorrect a medicine may not be dispensed or administered.
	If a patient asks a question about the medication prescribed by you or another prescriber do not guess the answer – check it using resources!	Incorrect information can cause patient harm, always stop to check if you are unsure.

Further reading

Department of Health, 1989. Review of prescribing, supply and administration of medicines. A Report on the supply and administration of medicines under group protocols. (Department of Health, April, London).

Royal Pharmaceutical Society 2016. A Competency Framework for all Prescribers. <http://www.rpharms.com/support-pdfs/prescribing-competency-framework.pdf>

Background

The General Pharmaceutical Council (GPhC) Standards outline the key skills and competencies that you must have attained in order to make you a safe and competent pharmacist and these have also been discussed in the introduction. Your MPharm degree must be progressive, dealing with issues in an increasingly more complex way until the right level of understanding is reached.

The GPhC Standards also require the integration of science into pharmacy practice. So what do they mean by integration? In plain terms, what we teach you in an MPharm degree must be linked in a coherent way so that you learn to appreciate how science is essential to contemporary pharmacy practice. It is critical that you develop a full range of skills and competencies integrated across all modules/components and all years.

MPharm programmes strive to develop teaching and assessment methods which help to prepare you for your future career as a pharmacist. Ideally a learning process based on integration provides content with context and results in improved retention of knowledge. Therefore, most MPharm programmes deliver teaching in an integrated manner, referring to commonly prescribed drugs and possible patient outcomes where appropriate. Your lecturers will signpost you to how knowledge and skills link across and above to other parts of the course. In order to help you integrate your skills and knowledge we must also assess in an integrated manner. Schools and departments of pharmacy are in the process of developing new assessment methods to do this. In Queen's University Belfast (QUB) Criterion Referenced Assessments (CRAs) have been developed as a competency-based assessment designed to test integration. The examples in this chapter refer to this type of competency-based assessment which are used in year 1 and year 2 of the MPharm programme at QUB. Your university may assess you using a variation of this method or indeed use a different name, for example OSCEs. Whatever the method used it is imperative that you develop your key skills throughout your course and you can use the example stations in this chapter to check your progress. We have included a topic guide and competency list for each station as in previous chapters. You can check this guide to see if you have covered the material in your course to date and are therefore able to complete the stations.

What is a CRA?

The CRA is a form of assessment that is derived from a specific set of clear outcomes or criteria. From this set of criteria/outcomes assessors and students can all make reasonably objective judgements with respect to student achievement or non-achievement of these outcomes. On the completion of a CRA station you will have simply met the criteria and passed or have failed to meet the assessment criteria.

Key aspects of a competent performance or attainment for a first-year student have been established. From this a set of minimum criteria have been developed and assessments are based around these criteria. For example, a student should be numerically competent i.e. be able to verify safety and accuracy utilising pharmaceutical calculations.

Preparation

You are not expected to learn and regurgitate large volumes of information for this type of assessment. Most competency-based assessments will provide relevant reference texts or resources where information can be found.

How to approach a CRA task station

- Each station will have a standard task sheet; read through the task carefully **twice.**
- All six stations will be centred on one patient with a specific health problem/need.
- A timer is projected at the front of the room and an announcement will be made 2 minutes before the end of each 10-minute station.
- At the end of the 10 minutes a buzzer will sound and you can move to the next station.
- Complete the task using the resources available on the table.
- At the written stations place your answer sheet in the box provided at the end of the 10 minutes.
- In the verbal stations there will be an assessor and a patient. Your task will involve the patients only and they will make themselves known to you at the start of the station.

How to use station resources

All of the resources you will need will be present at the station – remember if there is a resource at the station it most likely is needed to complete the task correctly! The resource could be a text book, some laboratory results, various sample formulations of a medicine, dispensed medication, a BP monitor, a peak flow meter or indeed a patient.

- All equipment will come with full and easy-to-follow instructions.
- All dispensed medicines and devices will come with the patient information leaflet (PIL) and these can be referred to when counselling a patient.

How to approach a calculation

During the first year of the MPharm you have been introduced to numeracy skills in many of the modules.

The numeracy skills tested in the CRA are no more demanding than what you have covered already and a calculator will be available at the station. However, it is good practice to complete a calculation initially without the use of a calculator (i.e. attempt to come up with at least an estimate of the answer and then check this with a calculator). Many clinical errors have involved the incorrect input of numbers or decimal places into a calculator – so use both!

How to have a consultation with a patient

There will be at least one station that involves an interaction with a patient. As part of your MPharm course you may have counselled using the Calgary-Cambridge model (see Figure 3.1). You can employ this again when counselling your patient at the verbal station. In the verbal station you should take time to prepare what you want to say and make notes on this beforehand.

How to counsel a patient on prescribed medication or devices

In the verbal station you may have to counsel a patient on prescribed medication. All prescriptions in level 1 CRAs will be legally and clinically correct as these areas will be covered later in the course. You will not need to clinically evaluate the prescription in the verbal station.

You will need to introduce yourself and check that you have the correct patient. You do this by asking for the patient's full name and address and then comparing this against your prescription.

Before counselling patients on their medicines, it is important to:

1. Prepare beforehand
2. Communicate appropriately, have a two-way conversation with the patient – initiate the session and gather information
3. Explain the medicines-related information (oral and/or written) and check with the patient if there are any questions
4. Conclude interview (thank the patient).

Initiating Communication can include:
'Hello my name is ..., and I am a first-year pharmacy student.'
Gathering information:
'Is this prescription for you? Can I just check that I have the right person? Can you please give me your full name and address?'
Or if, for example, a parent or representative is picking up the prescription:
'Can I check the patient details with you to make sure that this is the correct prescription?'
Providing Information:
The patient can be counselled in conjunction with the PIL.
'Thank you Mrs Jones – have you any questions you would like to ask me about (fill in drug(s) here)?'
Thank the patients for their time.

Some patients will be involved in managing their own care, for example an asthmatic may monitor their own peak flow results and record these in a diary. During a patient consultation they may refer to this type of monitoring.

Patient profile

The stations are all based around your patient, Mr. Luke Brady.

Mr Luke Brady is a retired joiner (62 years old) and he has been diagnosed with COPD (chronic obstructive pulmonary disease) 6 months ago. COPD is the name for a collection of lung diseases including chronic bronchitis, emphysema and chronic obstructive airways disease. People with COPD experience airflow obstruction and therefore suffer from shortness of breath. Breathing difficulties are caused by long-term damage to the lungs, usually because of smoking.

When you see the 'Buddy' sign you will need to pair up with a partner so that the partner can act out the role of the patient.

Level 1 Criterion-Referenced Assessment – Station A: Example 8.1

Please read the following information carefully. You have 10 minutes to complete the task.

Background

Mr Luke Brady is a retired joiner (62 years old) and he has been diagnosed with COPD (chronic obstructive pulmonary disease) 6 months ago. COPD is the name for a collection of lung diseases including chronic bronchitis and emphysema. People with COPD experience airflow obstruction and therefore suffer from shortness of breath. Breathing difficulties are caused by long-term damage to the lungs, usually because of smoking.

TASK

Mr Brady has developed an infection and has been admitted to hospital. Mr Brady's lung function and arterial blood gases were measured on admission to hospital.

The spirometry results show that:

Post-bronchodilator the FEV_1/FVC is < 0.7

FEV_1 % is 45.8%; 75% predicted.

1. Using the results given above and the GOLD document provided, state the severity of Mr Brady's disease state according to the guidelines.

In addition, arterial blood gas results revealed PaO_2 to be 65 mmHg, $PaCO_2$ to be 40 mmHg and pH 7.38.

2. Using the references provided decide if Mr Brady has any type of respiratory failure.

Props

Gold COPD: Global strategy for diagnosis, management, and prevention of COPD – 2016. Retrieved 23 March 2016 from http://goldcopd.org/global-strategy-diagnosis-management -prevention-copd-2016/ (page 14 provided).

Patient: Respiratory failure. Retrieved 23 March 2016 from http://www.patient.co.uk/doctor/ Respiratory-Failure.htm.

Table 8.1 Normal values and acceptable ranges of the ABG elements

ABG element	Normal value	Range
pH	7.4	7.35 to 7.45
PaO_2	90 mmHg	80 to 100 mmHg
SaO_2		93 to 100%
$PaCO_2$	40 mmHg	35 to 45 mmHg

Station A – Candidate answer sheet

Candidate name:		Date:	

COMPLETE ALL ASPECTS OF THIS ANSWER SHEET

Aspect to consider:

1. Using the results given above and the GOLD document provided, state the severity of Mr Brady's disease state according to the guideline.

2. Using the references provided decide if Mr Brady has any type of respiratory failure.

Topic

COPD

Interpreting arterial blood gas results

Competencies

GPhC competencies.

10.2.4 (c) Identify and employ the appropriate diagnostic or physiological testing techniques to inform clinical decision making

Level 1 Criterion-Referenced Assessment – Station B: Example 8.2

Background

Mr Luke Brady is a retired joiner (62 years old) and he has been diagnosed with COPD (chronic obstructive pulmonary disease) 6 months ago. COPD is the name for a collection of lung diseases including chronic bronchitis and emphysema. People with COPD experience airflow obstruction and therefore suffer from shortness of breath. Breathing difficulties are caused by long-term damage to the lungs, usually because of smoking

TASK

Following admission to hospital, a sputum sample for Mr Brady has been cultured and *Staphylococcus aureus* detected.

1. Is *S. aureus* a Gram-positive or Gram-negative organism?

Antimicrobial susceptibility data is performed using disc sensitivity testing and the results for the isolate are:

Antibiotic	Zone of inhibition (mm)
Ampicillin	35
Clarithromycin	24
Ciprofloxacin	12
Tetracycline	14

Continued

Level 1 Criterion-Referenced Assessment – Station B: Example 8.2—cont'd

2. Based on the British Society for Antimicrobial Chemotherapy interpretation of zone diameters, which antibiotics could you recommend for treatment and why?

Whilst reviewing Mr Brady's notes, you find out he is allergic to penicillin.

3. What antibiotic would you now recommend for Mr Brady and why?

Resources

Denyer SP, Hodges NA, Gorman SP, Gilmore BF: *Hugo and Russell's pharmaceutical microbiology*, ed 8. 2011, Wiley-Blackwell.

Table 8.2   BSAC MIC and zone diameter breakpoints for staphylococci (amended)

	Interpretation of zone diameters (mm)		
Antibiotic	R ≤	I	S ≥
Amikacin	10	16–18	19
Tobramycin	20	-	21
Ampicillin	25	-	26
Penicillin	24	-	25
Ciprofloxacin	17	-	18
Azithromycin	19	-	20
Clarithromycin	14	10–17	18
Clindamycin	22	23–25	26
Erythromycin	16	17–19	20
Doxycycline	30	-	31
Tetracycline	19	-	20

Key:
R = Resistance
I = Intermediate
S = Sensitive
BSAC – British Society for Antimicrobial Chemotherapy
MIC – Minimum Inhibitory Concentrations

Station B – Candidate answer sheet

Candidate name:		Date:	

COMPLETE ALL ASPECTS OF THIS ANSWER SHEET

Aspect to consider:

1. Is *Staphylococcus aureus* a Gram-positive or Gram-negative organism?

Station B – Candidate answer sheet—cont'd

2. Based on the British Society for Antimicrobial Chemotherapy interpretation of zone diameters, which antibiotics could you recommend for treatment and why?

3. What antibiotic would you now recommend for Mr Brady and why?

Topic

COPD

Interpreting antimicrobial resistance results

GPhC Competencies

10.2.4(c) Identify and employ the appropriate diagnostic or physiological testing techniques in order to promote health.

10.1(e) Demonstrate how the science of pharmacy is applied in the design and development of medicines and devices.

Level 1 Criterion-Referenced Assessment – Station C: Example 8.3

Background

Mr Brady is a retired joiner (62 years old) and he has been diagnosed with COPD (chronic obstructive pulmonary disease) 6 months ago. COPD is the name for a collection of lung diseases including chronic bronchitis and emphysema. People with COPD experience airflow obstruction and therefore suffer from shortness of breath. Breathing difficulties are caused by long-term damage to the lungs, usually because of smoking

TASK

Mr Luke Brady requires an antibiotic suspension to treat a chest infection. The suspension should contain 250 mg of the antibiotic per 5 ml.

1. How much antibiotic should a 100 ml bottle contain?

Mr Brady has been prescribed a dose of 500 mg every 12 hours for 7 days.

2. How much of the suspension would Mr Brady use in 7 days?

3. How many 70 ml bottles of suspension would be dispensed so that Mr Brady could complete the course?

A calculator is required for this exercise.

Station C – Candidate answer sheet

Candidate name:		Date:	

COMPLETE ALL ASPECTS OF THIS ANSWER SHEET

Aspect to consider:

1. How much antibiotic should a 100-ml bottle contain?

2. How much of the suspension would Mr Brady use in 7 days?

3. How many 70-ml bottles of suspension would be dispensed so that Mr Brady could complete the course?

Topic

COPD

Calculations

Competencies

GPhC Competencies

10.2.4.(C) Verify safety and accuracy utilising pharmaceutical calculations

Level 1 Criterion-Referenced Assessment – Station D: Example 8.4

Background

Mr Brady is a retired joiner (62 years old) and he has been diagnosed with COPD (chronic obstructive pulmonary disease) 6 months ago. COPD is the name for a collection of lung diseases including chronic bronchitis and emphysema. People with COPD experience airflow obstruction and therefore suffer from shortness of breath. Breathing difficulties are caused by long-term damage to the lungs, usually because of smoking.

Your task is based around the formulation of an antibiotic suspension for your patient Mr. Luke Brady. Mr Brady has difficulty swallowing. For this reason tablets are not suitable. A suspension has been requested instead.

Task

Complete all aspects of the **answer sheet** provided:

1. Explain why it is important that Mr Brady shakes the bottle prior to taking each dose.

2. The suspension contains *polysorbate 80*. What is the role of this excipient in this formulation?

3. Why is the suspension provided as a powder for reconstitution and not a ready-to-use suspension?

Resources

Prop A – Amoxicillin powder for reconstitution. Bottle labelled appropriately including 'to be used within 14 days'.

Prop B – Patient information leaflet for Prop A.

PIL: http://www.medicines.org.uk/emc/medicine/26166/PIL/Amoxicillin+125mg+5ml+-+250mg+5ml+Oral+Suspension+Sugar+Free+BP/

Prop C – Copy of pages relating to polysorbate 80 from the Handbook of Pharmaceutical Excipients.

Station D – Candidate answer sheet

Candidate name:		Date:	

COMPLETE ALL ASPECTS OF THIS ANSWER SHEET

Aspect to consider:

1. Explain why it is important that Mr Brady shakes the bottle prior to taking each dose of the medicine.

2. Why is the antibiotic provided as a powder to be reconstituted and not as the suspension?

3. The suspension contains Polysorbate 80. What is the role of this excipient in this product?

Topic
COPD
Pharmaceutics
GPhC competencies
10.1. (e) Demonstrate how the science of pharmacy is applied in the design and development of medicines and devices
10.2.3 (b) Apply pharmaceutical principles to the formulation, preparation and packaging of products

Level 1 Criterion-Referenced Assessment – Station E: Example 8.5

Background

Mr Brady is a retired joiner (62 years old) and he has been diagnosed with COPD (chronic obstructive pulmonary disease) 6 months ago. COPD is the name for a collection of lung diseases including chronic bronchitis and emphysema. People with COPD experience airflow obstruction and therefore suffer from shortness of breath. Breathing difficulties are caused by long-term damage to the lungs, usually because of smoking.

Task

Mr Brady will need a range of drugs to treat his COPD. Using the resources provided at your station and looking at the chemical structure of these drugs, answer the questions below.

Complete all aspects of the **answer sheet** provided:

1. Using the BNF provided what is the therapeutic application of these drugs?

2. Other than the aromatic group, which functional group is found in all three molecules?

3. Highlight the functional group (i.e. pharmacophore) which confers amoxicillin its pharmacological properties.

Below are given the chemical structures of three known drugs:

Amoxicillin

Sulfamethoxazole

Level 1 Criterion-Referenced Assessment – Station E: Example 8.5—cont'd

Ciprofloxacin

Resources

British National Formulary.

Patrick G: *BIOS Instant notes in organic chemistry*. Garland Science, Taylor & Francis Group, 2012.

Station E – Candidate answer sheet

Candidate name:		Date:	

COMPLETE ALL ASPECTS OF THIS ANSWER SHEET

Aspect to consider:

1. Using the BNF provided, what is the therapeutic application of these drugs?

2. Other than the aromatic group, which functional group is found in all three molecules?

3. Highlight the functional group (i.e. pharmacophore) which confers on amoxicillin its pharmacological properties.

Topics
COPD
Organic chemistry – functional groups in medicinal molecules.
GPhC Competency
10.1. (e) Demonstrate how the science of pharmacy is applied in the design and development of medicines and devices

👥 Buddy activity

Level 1 Criterion-referenced Assessment – Station F: Example 8.6

Please read the following information carefully. You have 10 minutes to complete the task.

Background

Mr Brady is a retired joiner (62 years old) and he has been diagnosed with COPD (chronic obstructive pulmonary disease) 6 months ago. COPD is the name for a collection of lung diseases including chronic bronchitis and emphysema. People with COPD experience airflow obstruction and therefore suffer from shortness of breath. Breathing difficulties are caused by long-term damage to the lungs, usually because of smoking.

The wife of Luke Brady (Mrs Brady) has come into your community pharmacy to collect his prescription. The prescription is for an antibiotic to treat a chest infection.

Task

Counsel Mrs Brady on how the antibiotic should be taken, considering the **prescription, the dispensed antibiotic suspension** and using the **reference sources provided**.

You must:

- Check that your prescription is for the correct patient

- Explain the directions for use

- Explain the most common side effects

- Ask the patient/patient's representative if there are any questions

The station supervisor will play the part of Mrs Brady – let the supervisor know when you are ready to speak with him or her.

Please submit your notes page to the examiner at the end of the CRA and do not forget to include your name on the form.

DO NOT write on or remove any of the materials provided.

Station props that would be provided

| Resources |
| Patient |
| Prescription |
| Dispensed prescription item |
| BNF |

Station F – Candidate notes page

| Candidate name: | | Date: | |

Use the space below to make any notes before you counsel the patient.

Pharmacy Stamp	Age	Title, Forename, Surname & Address
	62	Mr Luke Brady
	D.o.B	1 Castle Drive, Irvinestown
	05/12/1954	NHS number

Endorsements

Clarithromycin Oral Suspension

250 mg/5 mL

250 mg every 12 hours for 7 days

| Signature of Prescriber | Date |
| *SG Kyle* | Today's date |

For dispenser No. of Prescns on fom	Dr SG Kyle
	Main Street Surgery
	Irvinestown
	BT66 7JY

Figure 8.1 Prescription for Mr Luke Brady.

Station F – Notes to station patient

You are the wife of Luke Brady.

In case asked, your husband is 62 years old with a date of birth of **05.12.1954** and your address is **1 Castle Drive, Irvinestown.** Mr Brady has COPD and currently has a chest infection.

The candidate should show you the dispensed medication, refer to the patient information leaflet and verbally explain the relevant details including:

1. The **directions** i.e. that you will follow to give the medicine to your husband:

   • Two 5-ml spoonfuls twice daily (every 12 hours)

   • The need to space doses out evenly and complete the course

   • The need to shake the bottle prior to each dose

2. Discussion of **side effects,** including that this medicine may cause stomach upset

3. Give you an opportunity to ask **questions**

Station F – Patient actor's brief

If the candidate does not identify you, say...

'You know I'm Luke Brady's wife, don't you? Just want to be sure that this definitely is the medicine for my husband.'

If the candidate does identify you as Mrs Brady and your husband as Luke Brady and checks address (and/or DOB), say...

'That's me (if asked, our address is 1 Castle Drive, Irvinestown and Luke's DOB is 05/12/1954.'

If the candidate asks if you are aware why Mr Brady has been prescribed antibiotic, say...

'Yes, it is to treat my husband's chest infection.'

If the candidate asks you about any past medical history say...

'My husband has a bad chest, they call it COPD.'

If the candidate asks if he has any allergies, say...

'Not that I know of.'

If the candidate does not explain the dose clearly, say...

'I don't quite understand – can you explain that again?'

If the candidate does not mention potential side-effects, say...

'Does this medicine have any side effects?'

If they haven't mentioned to shake the bottle before each use, say...

'Is this one of the medicines that you have to shake before using?'

Topic
COPD
Dealing with prescriptions
Patient consultation (basic – level 1)
GPhC competencies
10.2.2. (c) Instruct patients in the safe and effective use of their medicines and devices
10.2.2. (d) Analyse prescriptions for validity and clarity
10.2.2. (g) Communicate with patients about their prescribed treatment

Level 2 Criterion-Referenced Assessment – Station A: Example 8.6

Background

Mr Brady is a retired joiner (62 years old) and he has been diagnosed with COPD (chronic obstructive pulmonary disease) 6 months ago. COPD is the name for a collection of lung diseases including chronic bronchitis and emphysema. People with COPD experience airflow obstruction and therefore suffer from shortness of breath. Breathing difficulties are caused by long-term damage to the lungs, usually because of smoking.

Task

Following a respiratory tract infection Mr Brady needs to increase his use of his corticosteroid inhaler. The following has been prescribed:

Beclomethasone dipropionate (Clenil Modulite®) 400 μg twice daily.

Consider this treatment and using the resources provided complete all aspects of the **answer sheet** provided:

The structure of beclomethasone dipropionate **is:**

Level 2 Criterion-Referenced Assessment – Station A: Example 8.6—cont'd

1. What is the molecular formula of beclomethasone dipropionate?
2. Redraw the structure and circle the key functionality which is responsible for the key characteristic infrared stretches of beclomethasone dipropionate in 3500, 1600, 1700, and 1750 cm^{-1}.

Resource

Table of infrared absorption frequencies

Table of infrared absorption frequencies

Functional group	Characteristic absorption(s) (cm^{-1})
Alkyl C–H Stretch	2950–2850 (m or s)
Alkenyl C–H Stretch	3100–3010 (m)
Alkenyl C=C Stretch	1680–1620 (v)
Alkynyl C–H Stretch	~3300 (s)
Alkynyl C=C Stretch	2260–2100 (v)
Aromatic C–H Stretch	~3030 (v)
Aromatic C–H Bending	860–680 (s)
Aromatic C=C Bending	1700–1500 (m,m)
Alcohol/Phenol O–H Stretch	3550–3200 (broad, s)
Carboxylic Acid O–H Stretch	3000–2500 (broad, v)
Amine N–H Stretch	3500–3300 (m)
Nitrile C≡N Stretch	2260–2220 (m)
Aldehyde C=O Stretch	1740–1690 (s)
Ketone C=O Stretch	1750–1680 (s)
Ester C=O Stretch	1750–1735 (s)
Carboxylic Acid C=O Stretch	1780–1710 (s)
Amide C=O Stretch	1690–1630 (s)
Amide N–H Stretch	3700–3500 (m)

m = medium intensity
v = variable intensity
s = strong intensity

Level 2 Criterion-Referenced Assessment, Station A – Candidate answer sheet

Candidate name:		Date:	

COMPLETE ALL ASPECTS OF THIS ANSWER SHEET

1. What is the molecular formula of beclomethasone dipropionate?

2. Redraw the structure and circle the key functionality which is responsible for the key characteristic IR stretches of beclomethasone dipropionate in the 3500, 1600, 1700, and 1750cm^{-1}?

Topic
COPD
Organic chemistry – analysis
GPhC competencies
10.1 (e) Demonstrate how the science of pharmacy is applied in the design and development of medicines and devices

Solutions

Station 8.1 – Mark sheet

Candidate's Name		Date	

Essential Assessment Criteria	Yes	No
Candidate identifies that the patient has moderate COPD.		
Candidate should state that Mr Brady does not have type 1 or type 2 respiratory failure. (Type 1 respiratory failure is assumed when PaO_2 is less than 60 mm Hg (8 kPa) (hypoxaemia) with a normal or low $PaCO_2$.)		

Recommendation (tick most appropriate term):	Pass	Fail

Assessor's comments:

Assessor's signature _____

Station 8.2 – Mark sheet

Candidate's Name		Date	

Essential Assessment Criteria	Yes	No
Candidate should state that *Staphylococcus aureus* is a Gram-positive organism.		
Candidate should highlight clarithromycin and ampicillin as zones of inhibition for these antibiotics are in the sensitive range.		
Candidate should recommend clarithromycin as this patient is penicillin allergic and cannot take ampicillin (a penicillin).		

Recommendation (tick most appropriate term):	Pass	Fail

Assessor's comments:

Assessor's signature _____

Station 8.3 – Mark sheet

Candidate's Name		Date			

Essential Assessment Criteria	Yes	No
Candidate correctly calculates that 100-ml bottle contains 5000 mg or 5 g.		
Candidate correctly calculates that the patient will use 140 ml of the suspension.		
Candidate correctly states that two 70-ml bottles will need to be dispensed.		

Recommendation (tick most appropriate term):	Pass	Fail

Assessor's comments:

Assessor's signature _____

Station 8.4 – Mark sheet

Candidate's Name		Date			

Essential Assessment Criteria	Yes	No
1. Candidate correctly states that suspensions settle due to sedimentation, and that shaking ensures accuracy and reproducibility of dosing.		
2. *Polysorbate 80* is a suspending agent (surfactant). It is used to help stabilise the dispersed phase (the drug granules). Surfactant hydrophilic/hydrophobic structure stabilises at the interface between dispersed phase and dispersion medium preventing aggregation and hence sedimentation.		
3. Provided as a powder to minimize instability caused by e.g. physical instability (sedimentation). Addition of water may lead to spoilage e.g. by microbial growth.		

Recommendation (tick most appropriate term):	Pass	Fail

Assessor's comments:

Assessor's signature _____

Station 8.5 – Mark sheet

Candidate's Name		Date		

Essential Assessment Criteria	Yes	No
Candidate identifies the class of compounds as antibacterials.		
Candidate identifies the functional group as being amines.		
Candidate identifies the pharmacophore as being a lactam.		

Recommendation (tick most appropriate term):	Pass	Fail

Assessor's comments:

Assessor's signature_____

Station 8.6 – Mark sheet

Candidate's Name		Date			
Assessment criteria (Essential in bold)				Yes	No
1. Introduce themselves including name					
2. Identifies that this is the correct patient using name and address from the prescription					
3. Explains the purpose of the discussion					
4. Establishes that patient has no allergies					
Rationale for the use of clarithromycin					
5. Explains or establishes that patient knows that antibiotic is being used to treat a chest infection					
Dosing schedule					
6. Two 5-ml spoonfuls					
7. Every 12 hours (twice daily)					
8. Space the dose evenly throughout the day. Keep taking this medicine until the course is finished, unless you are told to stop.					
9. Shake the bottle before taking					
Side effects					
10. Counsels on side effects listed in BNF/PIL – should include at least one of:					
• Nausea					
• Vomiting					
• Tummy discomfort					
11. Candidate uses lay language when explaining side effects: assessor to note medical jargon used by candidate					
12. Refers the patient to the written information provided (PIL)					
13. Any other valid point:					
14. Asks Mrs Brady if she has any questions					
15. Thanks Mrs Brady for her time					
Professional behaviour					

Recommendation (tick most appropriate term):	**Pass**	**Fail**

Assessor's Comments:

Assessor's Signature: _____

Station 8.7 – Mark sheet

Candidate's Name		Date	

Essential Assessment Criteria	Yes	No
1. $C_{28}H_{37}ClO_7$		
2 Alcohol, alkene, ketone, ester		

Recommendation (tick most appropriate term):	Pass	Fail

Assessor's comments:

Assessor's signature_____

Further reading

Denyer, S.P., Hodges, N.A., Gorman, S.P., Gilmore, B.F., 2011. Hugo and Russell's Pharmaceutical Microbiology, eighth ed. Wiley-Blackwell.

General Pharmaceutical Council (GPhC): Standards of initial education and training for Pharmacists. Retrieved 19 April 2013 from <http://www.pharmacyregulation.org/education/education-standards>.

Kurtz, S.M., Silverman, J.D., Benson, J., Draper, J., 2003. Marrying content and process in clinical method teaching: enhancing the Calgary-Cambridge guides. Acad. Med. 78 (8), 802–880.

Modernising the pharmacy curriculum: A report for the modernising pharmacy careers pharmacist undergraduate education and pre-registration training review team. Retrieved 19 April 2013 from <https://hee.nhs.uk/sites/default/files/documents/Pharmacist-pre-registration-training-proposals-for-reform.pdf>.

Patrick, G., 2012. BIOS Instant Notes in Organic Chemistry. Garland Science, Taylor & Francis.

Ratka, A., 2012. Integration as a Paramount Educational Strategy in Academic Pharmacy. Am. J. Pharm. Educ. 76 (2), 19.

Rowe, R.C., Sheskey, P.J., Quinn, M.E., 2012. Handbook of Pharmaceutical Excipients, seventh ed. Pharmaceutical Press.

Wolf, A., 2001. Competence-based assessment. In: Raven, J., Stephenson, J. (Eds.), Competence in the learning society. Peter Lang, New York, pp. 453–466 (Chapter 25).

Index

Printed and bound by CPI Group (UK) Ltd, Croydon, CR0 4YY

03/10/2024

01040411-0001